Advanced Praise for
The War on Informed Consent

"Dr. Thomas is one of those rare courageous people who dare to stand up to the establishment when they see strong evidence that the establishment's policies are dangerous, even when it might cost them their career. This book seamlessly weaves together Dr. Thomas's remarkable life story with much valuable information about the risk/benefit ratio for vaccines. A must-read for parents who face expanding government mandates that steadily erode our personal freedom of medical choice."
—Stephanie Seneff, PhD, author of *Toxic Legacy*

"When an industry like Big Pharma infiltrates and takes over every facet of potential control that should oversee it—Centers For Disease Control and Prevention, medical boards, state and federal legislators, main stream media—and even helps write the laws limiting parental rights and consent, it is no wonder that most pediatricians live in constant fear of having their medical careers taken from them for, of all things, actually listening to the concerns of the parents of their young and vulnerable patients.

Doctor Paul Thomas is one of the few remaining caring and brave pediatricians who not only listens to the parents' well founded concerns but also respects their wishes and more importantly, their rights. Instead of being praised, Dr. Thomas has been punished by the medical community, in this case the Oregon Medical Board, which seeks to silence all those who dare oppose the industry in which they operate as paid servants.

Jeremy Hammond is one of the few courageous journalists who swims against this current of unparalleled corruption and, in his excellent book, *The War on Informed Consent: The Persecution of Dr. Paul Thomas by the Oregon Medical Board*, Mr. Hammond exposes this Kafkaesque trial for all those who still have the freedom to think and decide for themselves."
—Rob Schneider, actor

"Un-coerced informed consent to medical procedures and the sanctity of the doctor-patient relationship are the two pillars of medical ethics that are being rapidly eroded by modern-day medical bureaucracy. Jeremy Hammond documents how this pervasive state of affairs has imposed dire consequences for a caring, ethical pediatrician who recognized that applying CDC vaccine recommendations indiscriminately was detrimental to some children in his pediatric practice and modified his care appropriately to achieve better health outcomes than the national average. This book is a must-read for any parent who wants to know what they are up against when making educated decisions in the best interest of their child's health or looking for a pediatric provider."

—**Tetyana Obukhanych, PhD, immunologist, immune science educator at Building Bridges in Children's Health, and author of *Vaccine Illusion***

"Jeremy R. Hammond's new book is a terrifying dissection of how the focus of modern medicine has shifted from individual well-being to compliance with the demands of a cynical and ruthless bureaucratic class exerting its muscle against the population, and gaslighting anyone who gets in the way. At the center of it is the political show-trial of Dr. Paul Thomas in Oregon—as with so many other show-trials (so reminiscent of the Soviet Union and Warsaw Pact of yore) the evidence is transparently false, as Hammond forensically demonstrates. For the perpetrators, of course, it barely matters; they simply intend to menace anyone else who is thinking of standing up against them. But it also begs the question what will happen if we do not stand up against this twenty-first century racketeering operation masquerading as science. This, unfortunately, is the story of our time."

—**John Stone, British editor of AgeofAutism.com**

"It was a typical Oregon February afternoon in 2015, when I walked into an overflowing state senate hearing room filled with hundreds of parents and by serendipitous chance, sat next to and met Dr. Paul Thomas. Both of us testified that afternoon on the importance of parents being the primary decision-maker on behalf of their children, and how the proposed bill would eliminate the right of parents to exercise informed consent by removing their ability to withhold consent. I started my testimony that day reciting the oft quoted warning from Benjamin Rush that medical freedom must be put in the Constitution to prevent medicine from forcing people to submit to only what the dictating outfit offers.

What the Oregon Medical Board is doing to Dr. Thomas is a fulfillment of that prophesy. Jeremy Hammond thoroughly explores and exposes how the state's medical licensing board, in disciplining Dr. Thomas, ignores scientific data, disregards and perverts existing laws which protect individual rights, and in the process, subverts the principles of liberty and freedom that were the foundation of the experiment in self-government that America is. If the Medical Board succeeds in upholding its suspension, we will be one step closer to a totalitarian era, where our bodies are truly owned by the state, and freedom and liberty are but an illusion."

—Robert M. Snee, JD, cofounder of Oregonians for Medical Freedom

"Jeremy Hammond's exposé on the persecution of Dr. Paul Thomas by the Oregon Medical Board is more than about the targeting of a single pediatrician. Hammond methodically lays bare what parents of vaccine-injured children have known for decades—the systematic violation of the ethical and legal right to informed consent by governments, medical professionals, and regulatory agencies.

The 'immediate danger to public health' is the intentional efforts to coerce consent by denying parents vaccine risk information and using threats to silence physicians from telling the truth that vaccines can and do cause harm.

The unfortunate reality is that the Oregon Medical Board is not a rogue board; rather they exemplify what has gone wrong with the medical profession. Hammond 'pulls back the curtain' and reveals the level of fraud, corruption, and malfeasance pervasive in medicine today.

Our right to informed consent is more than the foundation of ethical medicine. It is the very essence of liberty. When informed consent is denied, we are no longer free."

—Ted Kuntz, president of Vaccine Choice Canada

"In *The War on Informed Consent*, Jeremy Hammond systematically deconstructs numerous lies and ploys promoted by the allopathic establishment, showing how regulatory agencies and legislators have been captured, science has been corrupted, and children are being harmed. If you've ever wondered how a highly respected pediatrician such as Paul Thomas could be falsely portrayed as a villain, read this book. A compelling, well-documented exposé of the vaccine industry's subversive influence on the practice of medicine!"

—Neil Z. Miller, medical researcher and author of *Miller's Review of Critical Vaccine Studies*

"*The War on Informed Consent* tears down the manipulative and coercive dealings of a state medical board that is bullying a doctor for holding true to his oath to 'first do no harm' and for respecting his patients' rights to informed consent. The in-depth research and interview with Dr. Paul Thomas are indicative of the great investigative work of Jeremy R. Hammond."

—Wayne Rohde, author of *The Vaccine Court 2.0*

"If you want to understand why America's children are plagued with chronic illness despite an abundance of medical care, then you need to read this book that tells the journey of man wise enough to see, humble enough to admit he sees, and brave enough to do something about it. And then you'll want to join him."

—Bernadette Pajer, host of *An Informed Life Radio*,
Informed Choice Washington

"Jeremy Hammond does an amazing job of exposing the attack on informed consent by governmental health authorities. This book will make you think deeply, as it exposes the history of corruption, and the lack of real science supporting the benefits of large scale vaccination. If you are on the fence about vaccines . . . if you are looking to get more informed so that you can make an intelligent, science based decision, this book is a must-read."

—Dr. Peter Osborne, founder of Gluten Free Society and
bestselling author of *No Grain, No Pain*

"If you leave yourself a lifeline, then in time, when the going gets really rough, you will reach back and take it. Eventually, painfully you will come to the realization that that lifeline is as illusory as 'Safe and Effective.' Paul Thomas left himself no lifeline. He not only challenged the corporate medical business model in his day-to-day practice by daring to provide parents with informed consent and choice, but he dared to perform and publish his own vaccine safety science. Delivering on a peer-reviewed vaxxed versus unvaxxed study that unequivocally highlighted the adverse health consequences of vaccination, the system in rage and panic demanded the head of this 'turbulent priest.' Thomas was excommunicated. And the health freedom community—massive and growing—provided with a true hero. The lifeline is a shackle after all."

—**Dr. Andrew Wakefield, writer and director of** *Vaxxed:*
From Cover-Up to Catastrophe **and writer, director,**
and producer of *1986: The Act*

THE WAR
ON
INFORMED
CONSENT

THE WAR ON INFORMED CONSENT

THE PERSECUTION OF DR. PAUL THOMAS BY THE OREGON MEDICAL BOARD

Jeremy R. Hammond

Foreword by Robert F. Kennedy Jr.

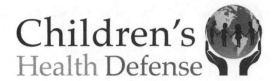

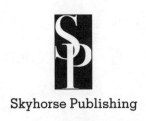

Skyhorse Publishing

Skyhorse Publishing books may be purchased in bulk at special discounts for
sales promotion, corporate gifts, fund-raising, or educational purposes. Special
editions can also be created to specifications. For details, contact the Special Sales
Department, Skyhorse Publishing, 307 West 36th Street, 11th Floor, New York,
NY 10018 or info@skyhorsepublishing.com.

Skyhorse® and Skyhorse Publishing® are registered trademarks of Skyhorse
Publishing, Inc.®, a Delaware corporation.

Visit our website at www.skyhorsepublishing.com.

10 9 8 7 6 5 4 3 2

Library of Congress Cataloging-in-Publication Data is available on file.

Print ISBN: 978-1-5107-6908-3
Ebook ISBN: 978-1-5107-6909-0

Printed in the United States of America

Contents

Foreword

by Robert F. Kennedy Jr.

I just ethically could no longer do business as usual, meaning the CDC's schedule, when I became very clearly aware of harm.

—Dr. Paul Thomas, MD

Dr. Paul Thomas, MD, an ethical and successful pediatrician, chose to follow his clinical observations, conduct genuine science, uphold his oath to do no harm, and enable his patients to exercise their right to make informed decisions about their own health care. In so doing, he has placed his professional career in the crosshairs of the corrupt and vicious machine known as the American public health establishment.

To help parents navigate the decision-making process when it comes to childhood vaccinations, Dr. Thomas and Jennifer Margulis, PhD, wrote the book *The Vaccine-Friendly Plan*, which presents an alternative approach to the one-size-fits-all schedule of the Centers for Disease Control and Prevention (CDC). Then the accusations started coming from the Oregon Medical Board.

When challenged by the board to provide peer-reviewed evidence from the medical literature to support his alternative approach, which is focused in part on reducing the cumulative levels of neurotoxic aluminum that children are exposed to from vaccines, Dr. Thomas rose to the challenge and together with research scientist Dr. James Lyons-Weiler published a study showing that, compared to children who were vaccinated according to variable schedules, the children born into his practice who remained completely unvaccinated had significantly less incidence of diagnoses and office visits for a broad range of health conditions.

The health outcomes that Dr. Thomas helped parents to achieve with his pediatric patients by recognizing the need for individualized risk-benefit analyses clearly demonstrate that his alternative approach is the correct one.

Among other remarkable outcomes, Dr. Thomas's published data show that being born into his practice is associated with a fivefold decreased risk of being diagnosed with autism compared to the general population of highly vaccinated children. *None* of the unvaccinated children included in the study were diagnosed with attention deficit hyperactivity disorder (ADHD).

"What really saves them," Dr. Thomas reasoned, "is you have to be very observant at every well-child visit, and you stop vaccinating if you see any problems." A quality assurance analysis of his clinical data validated his empirical observation that there were "massive increases in health problems in the highly vaccinated and a massive decrease in health problems in the unvaccinated. And it was undeniable."

Observing and caring for children rather than blindly following the unscientific mandates of the captured public health establishment has made Dr. Paul Thomas a modern iteration of Dr. Thomas Stockman in Henrik Ibsen's *An Enemy of the People.* While the enviable health outcomes shown by his data are indeed undeniable, this didn't stop the Oregon Medical Board, just days after his study was published, from frantically suspending Dr. Thomas's license on the demonstrably false pretext that his approach represents a threat to public health.

In exquisite detail, independent journalist Jeremy R. Hammond details the story of a heroic physician in *The War on Informed Consent: The Persecution of Dr. Paul Thomas by the Oregon Medical Board.* Hammond lays bare the twisted, corrupt, and biased prosecution of a doctor who put his patient's health first and who possessed the moral courage to speak truth to the corrupt and powerful. The forces aligned against Dr. Thomas seek to silence dissent as they promote an intolerable status quo that places the pharmaceutical industry's profits before children's health.

"We simply do informed consent," said Dr. Thomas in summarizing his alternative ethical approach. And for doing what should be done for *every* child, he has been pilloried in the mainstream press and attacked by the medical establishment. Although he knew that he would be risking his medical career by doing so, he chose to take a courageous stand and fight not only for his own pediatric patients, but for children everywhere whose parents are bullied into complying with a "standard of care" that rejects the need for individualized medicine and informed consent.

Hammond's work is of vital importance to the nation at a time when Americans are being bribed, sanctioned, and intimidated into submitting to COVID-19 vaccinations despite the absence of data on long-term safety and effectiveness. Every citizen should ask whether it is prudent to accept the dictates of public health authorities who claim the mantle of science and yet persecute those who do real scientific research that does not align with the political agenda of achieving high vaccination rates. Hammond is asking the reader to consider the evidence and question those who seek to sanction those who courageously tell the truth at a time when our nation is starving for honesty and for leaders who will place the interests of the people—and especially of children—above the political and financial interests of the pharmaceutical industry and the corrupt medical establishment.

Introduction

On December 3, 2020, the Oregon Medical Board issued an emergency suspension order to prevent renowned pediatrician Paul Thomas, MD, from seeing his patients by stripping him of his license.

The ostensible reason given by the board for this action against Thomas, who is affectionately known as "Dr. Paul" by his patients and peers, is that his "continued practice constitutes an immediate danger to public health".

Thomas is perhaps most well known as coauthor, along with Dr. Jennifer Margulis, of the book *The Vaccine-Friendly Plan*, which provides guidance to parents who want to protect their children from infectious diseases but have concerns about vaccines. The book is a bestseller and at the time of writing is showing a five-star rating from over 1,800 customer reviews on Amazon.

Since 2008, Thomas has practiced pediatrics out of his clinic, Integrative Pediatrics, which is in Beaverton, Oregon, within the metropolitan area of Portland.

The main accusation leveled at Thomas by the state medical board is that he has "breached the standard of care" in his practice by having many patients who are not vaccinated strictly according to the routine childhood schedule recommended by the Centers for Disease Control and Prevention (CDC).

The story the medical board tells is one of a reckless and "bullying" doctor who coerces his pediatric patients' parents *not* to follow the CDC's recommendations and whose gross negligence in this regard has caused harm to children and negatively impacted the health of the community.[1]

But that's not the true story.

The *true* story is that parents have flocked to Integrative Pediatrics precisely because they've been bullied, with the state's approval, by pediatricians in other practices who choose to dutifully serve the bureaucrats in government by compelling parents to strictly comply with the CDC's schedule.

Parents who *did* comply and then witnessed their children suffer harm as a result are mocked and derisively labeled "anti-vaxxers" for learning hard lessons from their firstborn children that they then apply to younger siblings by making different parenting choices. (Often, such parents respond to the derogatory label by insisting on being described as "ex-vaxxers," but government officials and the major media institutions refuse to hear them.)

Parents who *do* vaccinate their children, but not strictly according to the CDC's schedule, are also lumped into the group monolithically labeled "the anti-vaccine movement" by apologists for the one-size-fits-all approach of public vaccine policy.

These parents have all been told a million times that vaccines are "safe and effective." They are well aware of the arguments in favor of vaccinations that we all hear incessantly from government officials, medical professionals, and the mainstream media.

They are also perfectly familiar with the tale of how, in 1998, public enemy number one, Dr. Andrew Wakefield, published a fraudulent study in *The Lancet*, later retracted, claiming to have found an association between the measles, mumps, and rubella (MMR) vaccine and autism.[2] These parents know that numerous studies have since been published that failed to find an association.

They know that, by choosing to dissent from or criticize public vaccine policy, they are placing a target on their back. They know they will be met with disapproval by other members of their own family, accused of being irresponsible parents, scolded, and scorned. They know that they will be viciously attacked by government officials and policy advocates masquerading as journalists, as well as by doctors and other members of their community.[3]

And yet, despite the bullying and intimidation, they remain unmoved. There is one simple reason for this: *they see it as their duty as responsible parents to act in their children's best interest no matter what societal pressures are placed on them to conform with expected behavior.* Consequently, they do their own research, think for themselves, draw their own conclusions, and take a stand to protect their children.

In many cases in Portland, parents who face the scornful intimidation of a routine well-child visit at their pediatrician's office and still insist on exercising their right to make an informed choice *not* to vaccinate are told that they must either *comply* with the CDC's recommendations or *find another pediatrician.*[4]

And, so, they go to Dr. Paul.

With respect to the medical board's suspension order, Paul Thomas says he knew the moment *The Vaccine-Friendly Plan* was published that this day was coming. He knew at the time that, because he was challenging the CDC's schedule and therefore the "standard of care" of the medical establishment, he would be placing a target on his back and risking his career.

But he did it anyway.

Why?

The Oregon Medical Board wants us to believe it's because he's a villain who demonstrates reckless disregard and poses a danger to public health. The media have run with that story.

However, what neither the board's order nor the media has disclosed is that the board's suspension order was issued just eleven days after Thomas published a study in a peer-reviewed medical journal showing that, among the children born into his practice, those who remained completely unvaccinated were diagnosed at significantly lower rates than vaccinated children for a broad range of health conditions and disorders.

The difference in health outcomes was even more dramatic when Thomas and his coauthor, research scientist Dr. James Lyons-Weiler, looked at cumulative incidence of office visits for given diagnoses rather than incidence of diagnoses alone. This result strongly suggests that his vaccinated patients not only suffer from a higher rate of chronic health conditions, but also that their conditions are more severe, therefore requiring more frequent visits to his clinic.

The study is titled "Relative Incidence of Office Visits and Cumulative Rates of Billed Diagnoses Along the Axis of Vaccination." It was published in the *International Journal of Environmental Research and Public Health* on November 22, 2020.

As Thomas and Lyons-Weiler emphasize in the study, they do not show that vaccinations are the *cause* of the evidently worse health outcomes among vaccinated children. But what the results of the study *do* demonstrate to a reasonable degree of certainty is that his unvaccinated patients are healthier than vaccinated children and place *less* of a burden on the health care system.[5]

Importantly, this was peer-reviewed evidence that the medical board had *asked* Thomas to produce to support his practice of vaccinating patients according to the principles of his "vaccine-friendly plan."

Yet, when Thomas surmounted this challenge by obtaining Institutional Review Board (IRB) approval and publishing the deidentified data comparing health outcomes between vaccinated and unvaccinated children, the board's emergent response was to suspend his license until further notice "while this case remains under investigation"—and on grounds that are *completely belied* by the publicly available evidence.[6]

The real story here isn't one of a rogue doctor dismissing science and recklessly endangering his pediatric patients by bullying their parents into accepting "alternative" care. The real story is one of a rogue medical board dismissing science and recklessly endangering public health by encouraging pediatricians to bully their parents into strict compliance with the CDC's schedule and selecting Paul Thomas, MD, to set an example to other physicians of what their punishment will be if they instead choose to respect parents' right to informed consent.

But that story doesn't begin in December 2020. To tell the true story and fully appreciate its significance, we need to go back and review the sequence of events that led Paul Thomas to this pivotal moment in his life's journey.

A Young "Revolutionary" in Africa

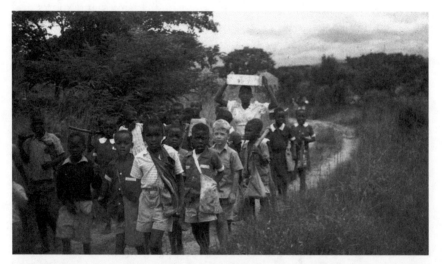

Paul Thomas grew up in the former British territory of Rhodesia, located in southern Africa where Zimbabwe is today *(photo courtesy of Paul Thomas).*

Paul Thomas was born in Portland, Oregon, on March 27, 1957, but he spent most of his childhood growing up in southern Africa. In 1961, his family moved to what was then the British territory of Rhodesia, which was located where Zimbabwe exists today on the northern border of South Africa.

One of four children of missionary parents, Paul and his family were the only white people living in the village of Arnoldine, where there was no running water or electricity. Paul and his sister Mary were the only white kids in the village school. While living in Africa, his parents also adopted five children.

In 1964, an opposition party named the Rhodesian Front declared independence, and its white leader, Ian Smith, was put in place as prime minister, a position that he held until 1979. The Republic of Zimbabwe was established in the place of Rhodesia in 1980. Smith was born in Rhodesia, but his party opposed any transition to democratic rule, which would mean the end of rule by a white minority. The regime he led was never internationally recognized.

In 1966, when it was discovered that Paul Thomas, who was nine years old, was attending the village school, he was removed to an all-white school in keeping with a policy of apartheid-like segregation. He developed two separate groups of friends: the white kids at the school and the black kids at home. At school, he excelled in academics and sports and was eventually selected as "Head Boy," an honor given to the top male student of the oldest grade.

In 1968, the breakaway regime held a ceremony to lower the Union Jack and raise the new Rhodesian flag in its place. At school, eleven-year-old Paul was expected to do the same in keeping with his duty as Head Boy. Considering the new government to be an unlawful regime, he courageously refused.

Two years later, Paul began attending high school at Waterford Kamhlaba in Swaziland, which had been established in 1963 as the first multiracial school in southern Africa. Among his schoolmates were daughters of Nelson Mandela, an anti-apartheid revolutionary who would go on to serve as president of South Africa from 1994 to 1999.

Although still a child, Paul Thomas, like Nelson Mandela, was deemed a threat by the powers-that-be. In 1973, at age fifteen, he was arrested by the Rhodesian government for distributing educational materials considered "revolutionary."

The Path of a Pro-Vaccine Pediatrician

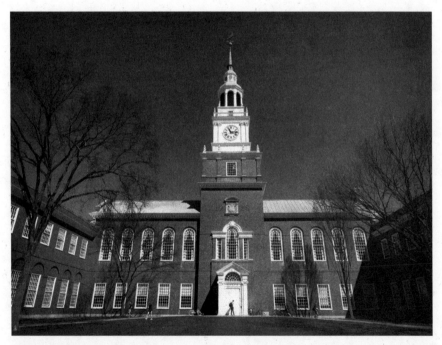

Dartmouth College Campus Library Building *(photo by David Mark, Licensed under Pixabay License)*[1]

In January 1974, Paul Thomas moved to Merced, California, to live with his aunt and uncle. He describes having experienced culture shock upon his return to the United States.

He took a job working as an orderly in a hospital until the fall of that year, when he entered his freshman year at Kalamazoo College in Michigan, where he studied premedicine. In 1975, he went back to California to study at the University of the Pacific, obtaining his Bachelor of Arts degree in biology in 1979. He continued his studies there and was a teaching assistant until 1981, when he obtained his Master of Science degree in biology.

From 1981 to 1985, he attended Dartmouth Medical School, an Ivy League institution in Hanover, New Hampshire, where he earned his degree as a Doctor of Medicine. From 1985 to 1987, Thomas completed the rigorous first two years of internship and pediatric residency at the Fresno location of the University of California, San Francisco (UCSF Fresno).

In 1986, Thomas adopted his first child, Natalie, at birth. His second child, Noah, was born the following year. From 1987 to 1988, Thomas continued his pediatrics residency at the University of California, San Diego (UC San Diego). In 1988, he moved back to Portland, Oregon, and worked as an attending physician at Emanuel Children's Hospital, where he also taught residents and medical students. In 1991, he married his current wife, Maiya, and in 1993, his third child, Tucker, was born.

That same year, Thomas joined Westside Pediatrics in Portland, a private group practice where he practiced alongside four other pediatricians.

In 1996, Thomas's fourth child and youngest son, Luke, was born. In 2000, Paul and Maiya became guardians of Aja, a girl the same age as Noah. Three years later, tragedy struck when Thomas's African sister, Tsitsi, died of congestive heart failure at the age of forty-three. She had moved to New Hampshire after the death of her husband and was the mother of four children: Zanele, an eleven-year-old girl; Themba and Tare, two boys aged twelve and fifteen, respectively; and Rufaro, who had reached adulthood and was attending college in another state. Paul and his wife took them in, bringing the number of children in the family to nine: three biological and six adopted.

"My kids are fully vaccinated, by the way," Dr. Thomas said in an interview with me. "So, I was still unaware of vaccine risk. This was back—you know, my youngest was born in 1996, and I just hadn't woken up yet."

"I come from a background of not being aware of vaccine risk," he explained. "I come from a background of being very well trained that vaccines are 'safe and effective.' I believed it."

Parents are told to listen to doctors and trust their ostensibly superior knowledge about vaccines, but doctors don't actually get much education about vaccines in medical school.

As Thomas related, "When you're in training in pediatrics, you don't get any training on vaccines while you're in school other than the diseases for which you vaccinate and how *horrible* they are and how wonderful it was that we had a vaccine. Alright, that's the extent of the education that we got in medical school."

He also said that when you get into residency, you don't have time to research things in depth on your own: "What you're learning at that point is learning what to do. You learn protocols, and so when it comes to how to vaccinate, you learn what the Academy of Pediatrics and the CDC want you to do—and that's what you do."

He was referring to the American Academy of Pediatrics (AAP), the trade organization that plays an important role in establishing the CDC's recommendations as "standard of care" in pediatric practices across the country.

"And honestly," Thomas continued, "for a long time—and I know most pediatricians still do this—you have the idea in your mind that, 'How could I, a lowly pediatrician who's just in training or just out of training—how could I know more than the CDC and the Academy of Pediatrics?' I mean, these are the best of the best who've risen to the top to give us this guidance, right? That's what we *think*. Well, that's what I *thought*."

That was before he became aware of the endemic corruption and conflicts of interest that exist within the medical establishment, of which government agencies like the CDC and FDA are an integral part.

That was before he started deeply researching the scientific literature for himself, in keeping with the advice of David Sackett, "the father of evidence-based medicine," who once quipped, "Half of what you'll learn in medical school will be shown to be either dead wrong or out of date within five years of your graduation; the trouble is that nobody can tell you which half—so the most important thing to learn is how to learn on your own."[2]

The Proven Untrustworthiness of Public Health Officials

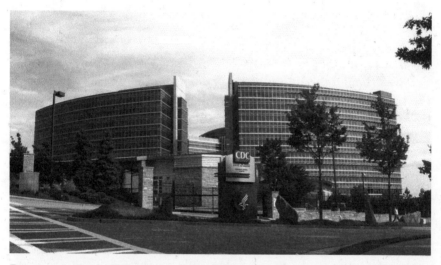

Entrance to the headquarters of the Centers for Disease Control and Prevention in Atlanta, Georgia *(Daniel Mayer/CC BY-SA 3.0)*[1]

When it comes to the subject of vaccines, parents across the country are incessantly bombarded with the message that they should *not* do their own research or think for themselves but instead simply trust public health authorities to determine what is in their child's best interests.

Parents are told to trust "the science," which is treated synonymously with whatever it is that public health officials proclaim. The trouble is that what government officials and the mainstream media *say* science says and what the science actually tells us about vaccines are two completely different things.

This is the reality of which those who do their own research are well aware, but it's a demonstrable truth that remains completely unacknowledged within the mainstream discourse.

Sometimes the cognitive dissonance within the medical establishment manifests itself glaringly. For instance, while government officials insist on one hand that vaccines are "safe and effective," it administers a program designed to effectively shift the financial burden for vaccine injuries away from the pharmaceutical industry and onto the taxpaying consumers.

This came about in the 1980s, while Thomas was attending medical school. Vaccine injury lawsuits against pharmaceutical companies were piling up, particularly for the diphtheria, tetanus, and whole-cell pertussis (DTP) vaccine and, to a lesser extent, the oral polio vaccine (OPV), which was responsible for causing every domestic case of paralytic polio in the US after 1979.[2]

Even though the risk of getting polio from the vaccine had become greater than the risk from the wild virus, and even though an alternative inactivated polio vaccine (IPV) was available, the FDA in 1984 declared that "any possible doubts, *whether or not well founded*, about the safety of the vaccine cannot be allowed to exist in view of the need to assure that the vaccine will continue to be used to the maximum extent consistent with the nation's public health objectives."[3] (Emphasis added.)

That neatly illustrates the attitude of public health officials today regarding the risks of vaccination: when the policy goal of achieving high vaccination rates conflicts with individuals' personal best interests and public health, it is the policy goal that takes precedence.

The way the *New York Times* tells the story, "anti-vaccination" groups began appearing in the country because parents saw a documentary aired by NBC in 1982 called *DPT: Vaccine Roulette*, which was "dangerously inaccurate" and falsely "purported" an association between the vaccine—variably abbreviated DTP, DPT, or DTwP—and "seizures". Due to the irrational and misinformed fears of parents who rejected the science, companies "stopped making vaccines" because it wasn't worth "the corporate headache."[4]

The reality is that parents who were concerned about the safety of the DTP vaccine were not the parents who were ignoring the science *but the ones paying attention to it.*

Far from their concerns being ungrounded and stories of vaccine injuries being mere "anecdotes," research was showing that the DTP vaccine was indeed associated with serious harms. The year *prior* to the release of that documentary, for example, a major study was published in the *British Medical Journal* (now *The BMJ*) that found a statistically significant association between the vaccine and "serious neurological illness" such as seizures and encephalopathy.[5]

Parents who had vaccinated their children because they were told it was "safe and effective" only to witness their children suffer serious adverse events and long-term harms *rightly* began questioning the public relations slogan, looking into the science for themselves, and learning the truth that the vaccine had never been adequately tested for safety and was the subject of considerable controversy within the scientific community.[6]

Today, it is *uncontroversial* that the vaccine was highly "reactogenic" and caused "significantly" more adverse reactions than the vaccine it was replaced with, which includes an acellular rather than a whole-cell pertussis component (abbreviated DTaP). As a systematic review published in the journal *Vaccine* in 2018 points out, the whole-cell vaccine was "crude" by comparison, and the switch was "warranted" by the reports of the vaccine causing relatively rare but serious injuries.[7]

While the DTP vaccine was phased out in the United States and other developed countries, it continues to be widely used in the developing world. The assumption made by public health officials, in the United States and elsewhere, has been that by reducing incidence of the three target diseases, the vaccine will reduce childhood deaths. The scientific evidence, however, does not support that assumption.

For one, the vaccine had no obvious impact on the population-adjusted mortality rate from pertussis in the United States, which had already been declining since well before the vaccine came into widespread use, as can be seen in the following graph created from the CDC's data.[8]

In fact, this is true for infectious diseases in general. As noted in the AAP's journal *Pediatrics* in a summary of vital statistics published in 2000, "vaccination does not account for the impressive declines in mortality" witnessed during the twentieth century. In fact, "nearly 90% of the decline in infectious disease mortality among US children occurred before 1940", before most vaccines were available to help explain it.[9]

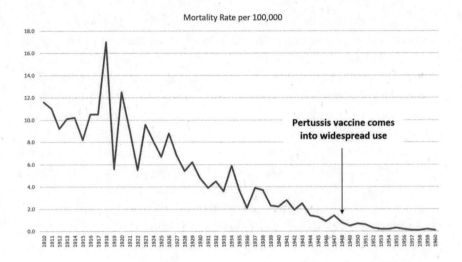

Mortality Rate per 100,000

Pertussis vaccine comes
into widespread use

Furthermore, even if a vaccine is effective at reducing mortality from the target disease, it doesn't necessarily follow that it will reduce overall mortality. This is because vaccines can have what are termed in the literature as "non-specific effects," meaning long-term effects other than those intended or anticipated and distinguished from acute adverse events that are temporally associated with vaccination.

Contrary to the assumption made by public health officials when introducing the DTP vaccine, studies done in recent decades have found it to be associated with an *increased* rate of childhood mortality.

As a study published in the *Lancet* journal *EBioMedicine* found, "DTP was associated with a 5-fold higher mortality than being unvaccinated."

As its authors remarked, "It should be of concern that the effect of routine vaccination on all-cause mortality was not tested in randomized trials. All currently available evidence suggests that DTP vaccine may kill more children from other causes than it saves from diphtheria, tetanus, or pertussis. Though a vaccine protects children against the target disease it may simultaneously increase susceptibility to unrelated infections."[10]

As the world's top researchers into the non-specific effects of vaccines noted in a *BMJ* article published in January 2020, the association between the DTP vaccine and increased childhood mortality is a consistent finding and is particularly pronounced among girls.[11]

The concern about vaccine trials not looking at long-term health outcomes, including mortality, is not limited to the DTP vaccine. *None* of the vaccines currently recommended by the CDC underwent randomized, placebo-controlled trials comparing *long-term* health outcomes, including all-cause mortality, between children who received the vaccine and children who did not.

The injury lawsuits against DTP manufacturers in the early 1980s incentivized the development of a less reactogenic product, which ultimately led to the DTP vaccine being phased out and replaced with the DTaP vaccine.

However, the US government had a solution in mind *other* than the development of safer and more effective means of reducing the burden of infectious disease. In fact, the government intervened in the market to effectively *eliminate* that key incentive for manufacturers to do so.

In 1986, the year that Paul Thomas adopted his first child, the National Childhood Vaccine Injury Act was passed into law. Because vaccine manufacturers were literally going out of business due to vaccine injury lawsuits and the increasing parental awareness that the safety studies conducted for licensure purposes were totally inadequate, the supply of vaccines was becoming unstable.

Complicating matters even further for the pharmaceutical companies was their difficulty in obtaining liability insurance due to the insurance industry's unwillingness to take on the risk.

Consequently, the public health policy goal of maintaining or increasing vaccination rates was threatened. To resolve that threat to public policy, the law granted broad legal immunity to manufacturers of vaccines recommended by the CDC for routine use in children. It also established the Vaccine Injury Compensation Program (VICP), which is funded by an excise tax on every vaccine dose administered.

The effect of the law is thus to shift the financial burden for vaccine injuries away from the pharmaceutical companies and onto the consumers—including those whose children are injured by vaccines.[12]

In 2011, the US Supreme Court upheld legal immunity for Big Pharma, judging that the "unavoidability" of vaccine injuries establishes "a complete defense" against lawsuits, provided that the vaccine was prepared according to specifications and accompanied with adequate warnings, which are found in the manufacturers' package inserts. In the Court's judgment, uniquely for the vaccine industry, "design defects" are "not a basis for liability."[13]

Policymakers characterized the law as being intended to benefit the public. That is certainly arguable, but what is incontrovertible is that it greatly benefited the pharmaceutical industry. The vaccine manufacturers were back in business, and the CDC continued adding more vaccines to its routine childhood schedule throughout the late 1980s and 1990s.

Helping the profit margins of the pharmaceutical companies even further was the artificial demand created by state laws mandating the use of their products as a requirement for school entry.

Included in many of those vaccines was a preservative called "thimerosal," which by weight is about half ethylmercury. While public health officials, the AAP, and the broader medical community continued to insist to parents that the CDC's recommended vaccines were "safe and effective," nobody had bothered to consider the long-term effects on children from the cumulative exposures to mercury they were receiving by following the CDC's schedule.

When the FDA finally got around to doing so, it was essentially by accident. In 1997, Congress passed the FDA Modernization Act, which included a provision requiring the FDA to compile a list of mercury-containing drugs on the market and the quantities of mercury contained in them. The FDA queried the industry, and the resulting list of products included numerous vaccines on the CDC's schedule.[14]

When researchers at the FDA's Center for Biologics Evaluation and Research (CBER) did the calculations in 1999, they found that the CDC's schedule was exposing infants to cumulative levels of mercury that exceeded the government's own safety guidelines. The finding that the levels exceeded the guidelines of the Environmental Protection Agency (EPA) was published by FDA researchers in the AAP's journal *Pediatrics* in 2001.[15]

Before it became public, health officials were panicked. The conundrum they were facing was elucidated in an email from Peter Patriarca, the director of the FDA's Division of Viral Products, to Martin Meyers, the acting director of the CDC's National Vaccine Program Office. If they were to call for the removal of thimerosal from vaccines, it would "raise questions about FDA being 'asleep at the switch' for decades". It would also "raise questions about various advisory bodies regarding aggressive recommendations for use."

People would naturally ask, "What took the FDA so long to do the calculations? Why didn't CDC and the advisory bodies do these calculations when they rapidly expanded the childhood immunization schedule?"[16]

At the same time, public health officials couldn't very well do *nothing* because, obviously, if they insisted that it was "safe" to continue exposing infants to such alarmingly high levels of mercury, it would *also* deservedly damage their credibility.

This concern was privately expressed by FDA researcher Leslie K. Ball, the lead author of the *Pediatrics* study, who observed that "toxicologists seemed reluctant to state any Hg [mercury] was 'safe,'" which opened government health officials to the criticism that they were "arbitrarily designating a certain level as acceptable when there continues to be so much uncertainty about the science in this area."[17]

In July 1999, the announcement was made that thimerosal would be phased out of most childhood vaccines, with manufacturers switching from multidose vials, for which they are required by the FDA to include the preservative, to single-dose vials.[18] Today, thimerosal is still used in multidose vials of influenza vaccine, which the CDC recommends be taken annually by everyone aged six months and up, including pregnant women.

To this day, the CDC self-contradictorily claims that its removal was simply "a precautionary measure", and that there's "no evidence of harm" from it. The CDC boldly asserts that ethylmercury from vaccines is "readily eliminated" from the body and so is "very safe".[19]

That claim, however, is belied by its own cited sources. A PDF document linked to on that page of the CDC's website cites six observational studies and an Institute of Medicine (IOM) review published in 2004 acknowledged the limitations of relying on observational studies in the absence of long-term randomized trials, described thimerosal as a "known neurotoxin", and acknowledged that ethylmercury from vaccines "accumulates in the brain" and "can injure the nervous system."[20]

On a Frequently Asked Questions webpage about thimerosal, the CDC says the same thing about the mercury in vaccines being "safe". That page links to another page providing a list of references.[21] The very first one is the 2001 *Pediatrics* study admitting that the CDC was responsible for exposing children to levels of mercury exceeding safety guidelines and whose lead author privately worried that it would be misleading to say it was "safe" given the scientific uncertainties.

In the published study, the researchers acknowledged that ethylmercury is toxic even at low doses and that it was possible that the exposure from vaccines could cause neurodevelopmental abnormalities in children.[22]

The second study the CDC cites on that page to support its claim that the mercury in vaccines is "safe" is a study published in *Environmental Health Perspectives* in 2005, which showed that ethylmercury is more readily eliminated from the blood but *more* persistent in the brain than methylmercury.

The authors also expressed concern that the toxicological properties of ethylmercury had not been sufficiently studied, requiring the government to adopt the scientifically invalid practice of basing its risk assessments instead on the toxicology of methylmercury.

They expressed the further concern that mercury in the brain was associated with "an active neuroinflammatory process" that had in turn been "demonstrated in brains of autistic patients".

Far from concluding that the mercury in vaccines is safe, they emphasized that studies were "urgently needed" to determine "the potential developmental effects of immunization with thimerosal-containing vaccines in newborns and infants."[23]

These are studies that the CDC cites to try to *support* its claims, to say nothing of studies that the CDC simply ignores. Naturally, to support the assertion that the mercury in vaccines is "safe" and that there's "no evidence" of toxicity at levels children have been exposed to from the schedule, the CDC does not cite, for example, a review on thimerosal published in *Neurochemical Research* in 2011 observing that all the studies reviewed had found evidence of neurotoxicity, which together constituted "unequivocal evidence" that ethylmercury "can affect neural tissues and functions" at "low doses" relevant to vaccines, making it "a likely risk factor for neurodevelopmental delays". [24]

Furthermore, *no* studies had been done to examine the synergistic toxicity of thimerosal being administered concomitantly with vaccines containing aluminum adjuvants, "which are also neurotoxic."

Given what is known from the available data, "it is reasonable to expect biological consequences in terms of neurodevelopment in susceptible infants." Studies to evaluate the health consequences of continued use of thimerosal in vaccines, including in developing countries, were "urgently" needed, and its use "should be reconsidered by public health authorities, especially in those vaccines intended for pregnant women and children."[25]

It would be superfluous to list more examples of how the CDC *willfully deceives the public* about the safety of vaccines.

Unbeknownst to Paul Thomas at the time, what many parents across the country had been discovering for themselves, oftentimes painfully, is that public health officials and other "experts" entrusted with determining the "standards of care" by which doctors practice medicine *are demonstrably unworthy of our trust.*

"We just didn't realize," Thomas explained, with respect to his time spent in medical school and pediatric residency, "that to rise to the top and sit on the committees that make the recommendations, you absolutely have to follow and say the right things. I mean, if you ever have anything in your background that questions vaccine safety or vaccine effectiveness, you don't get to move up. So it's a process that just pulls together the best speakers for the slogan—I mean the marketing slogan of 'safe and effective.'"

To arrive at where he is today in terms of knowledge, Thomas had to be willing to *question* everything he had ever learned about vaccines. More than that, as a pediatrician, he had to be willing to acknowledge the possibility that *something he was doing to children* with the intent of helping them *was instead causing them harm.*

This is evidently a rare quality among doctors, and Dr. Thomas's experience with the Oregon Medical Board goes some way toward helping to explain why.

The Endemic Corruption within the Medical Establishment

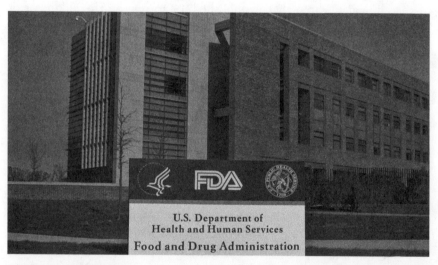

The FDA building where the agency's Center for Drug Evaluation and Research division is located *(US Food and Drug Adminstration/Public Domain)*[1]

When it comes to the topic of vaccines, the media goes so far as to dismiss any talk of "medical malfeasance, coverups, and corruption" as "misinformation" and "conspiracy theory." *Serious* discussion about public vaccine policy in the mainstream media is practically nonexistent.[2]

Yet the fact that endemic corruption exists within the medical establishment is not at all controversial within the scientific community. As a very widely cited paper published in *PLOS Medicine* in 2005 noted, conflicts of interest in medical research are "very common". Rather than majority expert opinion representing scientific truths, study findings "may often be simply accurate measures of the prevailing bias."

Scientists, policymakers, and medical practitioners are blinded by their own confirmation bias, grasping onto whatever information supports their preexisting beliefs while ignoring whatever does not. The peer-review process of medical journals served frequently "to perpetuate false dogma". Furthermore, "empirical evidence on expert opinion shows that it is extremely unreliable."[3]

In a *New York Review of Books* article in 2004, *Lancet* editor Richard Horton acknowledged that peer-reviewed journals had "devolved into information-laundering operations for the pharmaceutical industry."[4]

In the same magazine in 2009, *New England Journal of Medicine* editor Marcia Angell wrote, "It is simply no longer possible to believe much of the clinical research that is published, or to rely on the judgment of trusted physicians or authoritative medical guidelines."[5]

In a *Lancet* article published in 2015, Horton again lamented how "science has taken a turn towards darkness", in which "poor methods" were accepted because they "get results". "The apparent endemicity of bad research behaviour", he wrote, "is alarming. In their quest for telling a compelling story, scientists too often sculpt data to fit their preferred theory of the world. Or they retrofit hypotheses to fit their data. Journal editors deserve their fair share of criticism too. We aid and abet the worst behaviours."[6]

"To serve its interests," a study published in the *European Journal of Clinical Investigation* in 2013 concluded, "the industry masterfully influences evidence base [*sic*] production, evidence synthesis, understanding of harms issues, cost-effectiveness evaluations, *clinical practice guidelines* and healthcare professional education and also exerts direct influences on professional decisions and health consumers."[7] (Emphasis added.)

A good example of how the industry exerts influence on government policymaking is provided by the HPV vaccine. As detailed in a paper published in the *American Journal of Public Health* in 2012, "Merck promoted school-entry mandate legislation by serving as an information resource, lobbying legislators, drafting legislation, mobilizing female legislators and physician organizations, conducting consumer marketing campaigns, and filling gaps in access to the vaccine. Legislators relied heavily on Merck for scientific information."[8]

The CDC's role in deceiving the public about the science is acknowledged in the published literature, too. Referring to a CDC document outlining the rationale for its universal flu shot recommendation, a systematic review of the scientific evidence published in 2010 blasted policymakers for deliberately mischaracterizing the science to support its policy. The review authors remarked how policymakers within the CDC "do not weight interpretation by quality of the evidence, but quote anything that supports their theory."[9]

In a *BMJ* article published in 2015, associate editor Jeanne Lenzer observed how the CDC includes a disclaimer with its recommendations that it has no financial interests or other relationships with the manufacturers of commercial products, but how that isn't true because the CDC in fact receives millions of dollars in funding from the pharmaceutical industry through an organization called the CDC Foundation.[10]

In its own words, the CDC Foundation is "an independent nonprofit and the sole entity created by Congress to mobilize philanthropic and private-sector resources to support the Centers for Disease Control and Prevention's critical health protection work."[11] The foundation's partners include pharmaceutical companies AstraZeneca, Bayer, Eli Lilly, GlaxoSmithKline, Johnson & Johnson, Merck, Novartis AG, Novavax, Sanofi Pasteur, and Wyeth, among a long list of others.[12]

The US Congress has also acknowledged that parents' increasing lack of trust in public health officials is not without just cause.

In a June 2000 report, the House of Representatives' Committee on Government Reform excoriated the CDC and FDA for endemic conflicts of interest. At the CDC, waivers from conflict-of-interest rules were routinely granted to every member of its Advisory Committee on Immunization Practices (ACIP). The chairman of the committee had owned shares of stock in the pharmaceutical giant Merck, which manufactures numerous vaccines recommended by the CDC.

Of the eight committee members who voted to approve guidelines for the rotavirus vaccine in June 1998, half "had financial ties to pharmaceutical companies that were developing different versions of the vaccine." Of the five members of the FDA advisory committee who voted to approve the rotavirus vaccine in December 1997, three likewise had financial ties to companies developing different versions of the vaccine.

A particularly salient example of the corruption is Dr. Paul Offit, who joined the CDC's advisory committee in October 1998 and voted three times in favor on decisions related to the rotavirus vaccine, including the vote to add it to the Vaccines for Children (VFC) program, which makes vaccines available at no cost to low-income families through Medicaid. Concurrently, Offit shared ownership with the Children's Hospital of Philadelphia (CHOP) of a patent for the rotavirus vaccine being developed under a grant from Merck.[13]

Offit sat on the CDC committee until June 2003. Merck's rotavirus vaccine was licensed in 2006 under the trademark RotaTeq. The hospital sold its stake in the patent in 2008 for $182 million. Offit profited handsomely, publicly acknowledging that the deal made him "several million dollars, a lot of money". As he told *Newsweek*, the "small percentage" he received of the total was "like winning the lottery."[14]

Offit also happens to be one of the media's go-to experts on vaccines. In 2015, he wrote an op-ed in the *New York Times* accusing parents who choose not to vaccinate of *child abuse* on the grounds that Jesus, were he walking on Earth with us today, would advocate forcibly vaccinating children against their parents' will.[15]

The first FDA-licensed rotavirus vaccine that the CDC recommended for routine use in children was Wyeth's RotaShield. That vaccine was withdrawn from the market in 1999 because it was found to be causing intussusception, an often excruciating and potentially fatal condition in which part of the intestine telescopes in on itself. The FDA had approved RotaShield as "safe" despite clinical trials having shown an increased incidence of intussusception in vaccinated infants.

This finding was dismissed as "probably due to chance" by the FDA's Vaccines and Related Biological Products Advisory Committee (VRBPAC)—an unsurprising judgment given the financial conflicts of interest of most of its members.[16]

The US government itself, through the National Institutes of Health (NIH), developed, patented, and licensed technology to Wyeth for use in its rotavirus vaccine.[17] Another example of a pharmaceutical product for which the government patented and licensed technology is Merck's human papillomavirus (HPV) vaccine.[18]

Tellingly, when the FDA instructed Wyeth on which specific adverse events it should focus in postmarketing safety studies, *the risk of intussusception was not among them*. Researchers monitoring public postmarketing surveillance data, however, nevertheless picked up on reports of the adverse event, and studies were conducted that confirmed the association, which the CDC acknowledged as "a strong causal relationship".[19]

With no shortage of irony, government health officials uphold the story of RotaShield as a shining example of how the bureaucracies charged with ensuring vaccine safety are highly effective at doing so.[20]

Just as tellingly, when the CDC's advisory committee voted to *withdraw* its recommendation for routine use of RotaShield, Paul Offit suddenly found a conscience and *abstained* on the grounds that there would be "a perception of conflict" for him to vote against Wyeth's product while he was working on a competitor's vaccine.[21]

At the time of this writing, Paul Offit is a member of the FDA's vaccine advisory committee responsible for recommending COVID-19 vaccines to be authorized for emergency use while prelicensure trials remain underway.[22]

A Senate report in June 2007 blasted the CDC for seeking ever-increasing levels of funding year after year but having little to show for its exorbitant spending in the way of improved public health. Part of the problem was the "revolving door" by which CDC officials or contractors find lucrative ways to make their CDC connections pay off in the private sector. Exemplifying this problem was the CDC director herself, Julie Gerberding, under whose leadership bonuses for those in management increased dramatically, including a tenfold rise in the share of premium bonuses given to those within her office.[23]

Gerberding left her CDC job in 2009 and joined Merck in 2010 as president of its $5 billion global vaccine division. Merck's chief executive officer understandably described her as "the ideal choice".[24] In 2015, she sold shares of Merck worth over $2.3 million.[25] She is presently the chief patient officer and executive vice president of the company. Among her responsibilities is "strategic communications," which is essentially to say that she is now in charge of Merck's propaganda efforts.[26]

A 2009 report from the Office of the Inspector General for the Department of Health and Human Services, under which both the CDC and FDA operate, found that there was "a systemic lack of oversight" at the CDC with its ethics program for special government employees—such as the people who sit on its vaccine advisory committee. Nearly all financial disclosure forms for such employees were completed improperly. Only 3 percent of forms contained no omissions, and 64 percent of employees with one or more omissions were found to have potential conflicts of interest that the CDC had either failed to identify or failed to resolve.[27]

In January 2018, CDC Director Brenda Fitzgerald was forced to resign after it was reported that she had purchased tens of thousands of dollars in corporate stocks, including shares in a global tobacco giant and in Merck.[28]

In June 2019, vaccine manufacturer Pfizer announced that former FDA Commissioner Scott Gottlieb had joined its board. Known for having pushed for reforms under the Donald Trump administration to hasten the drug-approval process, Gottlieb remarked that joining Pfizer "uniquely positioned" him to advance "public health"—the usual euphemism for the pharmaceutical industry's financial interests.[29]

Just as the government has an incestuous relationship with and serves the interests of the pharmaceutical industry, so, too, does the American Academy of Pediatrics (AAP). As CBS News reported in 2008, "The vaccine industry gives millions to the Academy of Pediatrics for conferences, grants, medical education classes and even helped build their headquarters."[30]

As the 2007 Senate report noted, the CDC has manifestly failed in its ostensible mission to better public health. A study published in 2011 in *Academic Pediatrics* estimated that at least 43 percent of children had at least one chronic health condition. When children who were overweight, obese, or at risk for developmental delays were included, the figure rose to 54 percent.[31]

Among the conditions that have increased in prevalence are a broad range of autoimmune diseases, which is attributed to environmental factors that the CDC says it is at a loss to identify.[32]

Perhaps it is not really such a great mystery, given the aggressive use in developing infants and toddlers of pharmaceutical products specifically intended to permanently alter the functioning of their immune system.

The Absence of Studies Examining the Safety of the CDC's Schedule

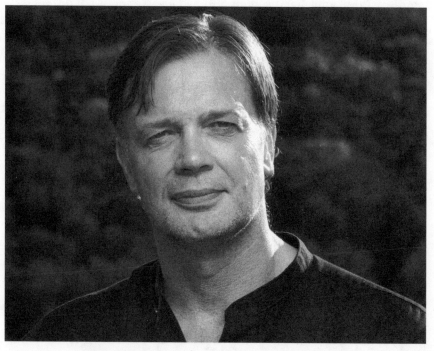

Andrew Wakefield *(courtesy of Andrew Wakefield)*

In 1998, *The Lancet* published a study written by Dr. Andrew Wakefield and twelve coauthors that has come to be regarded with infamy. The mainstream media refer to it almost obligatorily in articles discussing the topic of vaccines. The way the media present it, this study fraudulently claimed to have found a causal association between the measles, mumps, and rubella (MMR) vaccine and autism, and the belief that vaccines might contribute to the development of autism had its origins in that fraudulent claim.

However, that dominant mainstream narrative is false.

To start with, Wakefield and his coauthors did *not* claim to have found an association between the vaccine and autism. On the contrary, they explicitly stated that they did *not* show a causal link and concluded that studies should be done to determine *whether* there is an association.

The study was a case series, which is a type of study presenting clinical data about patients for the purposes of presenting findings that raise questions and proposing hypotheses to be explored with further research. The main finding of this case series was that twelve children who experienced regressive developmental disorders also had a gastrointestinal disorder.[1]

Today, the connection between gut disorders and autism is well established, with much research now focusing on questions such as the role of the gut microbiome in relation to neurological disorders.[2] But at the time their case series was published, Wakefield was pioneering research into this area. Nevertheless, he and his coauthors are not remembered for driving research into the gut-brain connection. Instead, Wakefield is singled out for vilification, and his coauthors are forgotten, as though he were the sole author of the study.

The Lancet retracted the article in 2010, over a decade after it was published and in response to the General Medical Council (GMC) in the United Kingdom having stripped Wakefield and his coauthor John Walker-Smith of their medical licenses. Walker-Smith was the gastroenterologist who examined the children and the senior author listed on the study (in the literature, the first author listed may be the primary but not the *senior* author, whose name is typically listed *last*).

The reason stated for the retraction was *not* that the paper had been found to be based on fraudulent data. Rather, the GMC had judged that the authors falsely stated that the children were "consecutively referred" and that their investigation with these children was not approved by the local ethics committee.[3]

The GMC had found Wakefield and Walker-Smith guilty not of fraud but "professional misconduct". What the mainstream media never tell the public, despite bringing up the study incessantly, is that Walker-Smith *appealed* the GMC's decision and *won*. He was reinstated in 2012 on the grounds that the GMC's charges against him were "untenable" and unsupported by the evidence.

The children were indeed consecutively referred according to the authors' plainly intended meaning of having been "referred successively, rather than as a single batch". Furthermore, *they did not require ethics approval for the procedures the children underwent under Walker-Smith's care because the procedures were clinically indicated for diagnostic purposes.* In some of the children, this process of clinical diagnosis led to treatment resulting in marked improvement of symptoms.[4]

The reason Wakefield did not join his colleague in appealing the GMC's ruling is that the legal costs were not covered by his insurance carrier.[5]

Where the MMR vaccine comes in is that Wakefield and his coauthors noted in their paper that *the parents* had associated their children's developmental regression with vaccination. That was the only "link" between the vaccine and autism discussed in the paper: the authors noted parents' concerns, *hypothesized* that there *might* be an association, and called for further research into this question.[6]

The claim that parental concerns about vaccines causing autism originated with the *Lancet* paper is consequently also false. Those concerns preexisted the clinical investigation of the twelve children included in the case series. In fact, the Institute of Medicine had issued a report *in 1991* discussing widespread parental concerns that vaccines might be causing autism.

The IOM found "no evidence" to support a causal relationship between the DTP vaccine and autism, which was unsurprising since, as the IOM also observed, no studies had been done to test that hypothesis.[7]

To many parents around the country, Andrew Wakefield is seen not as a villain but a hero, both for his role in pioneering research into the gut-brain connection in autistic patients and for directing attention to the potential role of vaccines in the rising incidences of a vast array of chronic diseases and developmental disorders.

We're told incessantly by the government, media, and medical professionals that the vaccine-autism hypothesis has been scientifically disproven. However, that is *false*.

To illustrate, we need only turn to the CDC's webpage on which it boldly declares that "Vaccines do not cause autism."[8] Naturally, since the CDC is *responsible* for the health outcomes in children caused by adherence to their recommended vaccine schedule, *there is an institutionalized incentive to find these products harmless,* and this confirmation bias is evident on the page.

To support its claim, the CDC cites observational studies and a review by the Institute of Medicine in 2004 that described the hypothesis as "biologically plausible", described thimerosal as a "known neurotoxin" that "accumulates in the brain" and "can injure the nervous system", concluded that the vaccine-autism hypothesis *cannot* be excluded on the basis of existing observational studies, and explicitly acknowledged *that none of the studies were even designed to test the hypothesis that vaccines can cause autism in genetically susceptible individuals.*[9]

The CDC also cites an IOM review in 2011 that again acknowledged that existing observational studies were inadequate to reject the hypothesis, and that researchers—including those from the CDC—were still failing to take into consideration the possibility of genetically susceptible subpopulations. Indeed, the CDC, by declaring that "Vaccines do not cause autism", is *rejecting* the standards of evidence adopted by the IOM and its conclusion that observational studies are insufficient to either *establish* or *reject* a causal association.

Instructively, this is a standard of evidence we *are* often reminded of when observational studies *do* find an association between vaccines and harm, in which case we are reminded that correlation does not necessarily mean causation. This is only forgotten when studies fail to find an association, in which case they are upheld as scientific proof of no link—even though, as the IOM rightly observed, "absence of evidence isn't evidence of absence", and observational studies have inherent methodological limitations that give rise to selection biases due to the lack of randomization and inability to control for countless confounding factors.[10]

An example of an important selection bias often described as "healthy user" bias comes from a study published in *JAMA* in 2015 that was widely misreported as having once again proven that there is no association between the MMR vaccine and autism *even among genetically susceptible children.* However, that conclusion does *not* follow from the study's findings.

On the contrary, what the study actually found was a *negative* correlation between vaccination and incidence of autism diagnoses among children who have an older sibling with autism. The authors did *not* attribute this to a protective effect of the vaccine. Rather, they observed that *the MMR vaccination rate among these younger siblings was lower.* Hence, what their study truly revealed is a healthy user bias that is not accounted for in other studies ostensibly intended to test the hypothesis. It's not that children with autistic older siblings were less likely to develop autism if they were vaccinated; *it's that that parents of an older child with autism are less likely to do the MMR vaccine with later-born children.*

In other words, the negative association can be explained by the fact that children in the study considered to be at highest risk of developing autism due to genetic susceptibility were pooled disproportionately into the "unvaccinated" group (which term, in this study, could mean they received all the recommended vaccines except the MMR).[11]

Subsequent studies also hailed by the media as once again disproving the hypothesis continued to *fail* to account for this healthy vaccinee selection bias.[12]

Studies to date have also focused on the MMR vaccine and thimerosal, even though the use of aluminum as an "adjuvant" in vaccines is of major concern to parents. Like ethylmercury, *aluminum is a known neurotoxin that can be transported by immune cells from the vaccination site through the blood-brain barrier and into the brain, where it accumulates.*[13]

In fact, this is acknowledged in the key study cited by the CDC to support its claim that aluminum from vaccines "is not readily absorbed by the body".[14]

Other studies have also pointed out numerous concerning flaws in that key study and the reasoning used by its authors to arrive at the evidently desired conclusion. For example, it is scientifically invalid to determine the effects of aluminum *injected* into *human* children based on a study of aluminum *ingested* by *rodents.*

The differing routes of entry are important because less than 1 percent of *ingested* aluminum is absorbed into the body.[15] By contrast, as the FDA itself observes, "parenterally administered drug products containing aluminum bypass the protective mechanism of the gastrointestinal tract . . . and it is deposited in human tissues."[16]

Studies support the biological plausibility of the hypothesis that aluminum-containing vaccines administered according to the CDC's schedule contribute to the development of autism in susceptible children. Like mercury, aluminum is associated with a neuroinflammatory process observed in children with autism.[17]

Of course, parents have a broad range of concerns about the health impact of vaccines other than the fear that they may contribute to the development of autism, and while they are told that science has proven that it's "safe" to vaccinate according to the CDC's schedule, concerned parents know that this is untrue.

For instance, for the purpose of persuading parents that they should strictly comply with the CDC's schedule, the *Washington Post* brazenly lies that "No new immunization is added to the schedule until it has been evaluated both alone and when given with the other current immunizations."[18] That is categorically *false*.

The truth is that, as acknowledged in an IOM review published in 2013, "No studies have compared the differences in health outcomes . . . between entirely unimmunized populations of children and fully immunized children." The IOM reiterated that "existing research has not been designed to test the entire immunization schedule" and, again, that "studies designed to examine the long-term effects of the cumulative number of vaccines or other aspects of the immunization schedule have not been conducted."

"Key elements" of the CDC's schedule that "have not been systematically examined in research studies", the IOM noted, included "the number, frequency, timing, order, and age at the time of administration of vaccines".

There was also limited and inadequate research into "health outcomes in potentially susceptible subpopulations of children who may have an increased risk of adverse reactions to vaccines (*such as children with a family history of autoimmune disease or allergies or children born prematurely*)". (Emphasis added.)

To resolve the uncertainties arising from the lack of research into the cumulative effects of vaccinating children according to the CDC's schedule, the IOM recommended that the US Department of Health and Human Services "incorporate study of the safety of the overall childhood immunization schedule into its processes for setting priorities for research".[19]

The author of the *Washington Post* article, Lena Sun, and the editorial board were informed of their error but refused to publish a correction—thus choosing to go on *willfully* deceiving parents in service to the government and, by extension, the pharmaceutical industry.[20]

In another illustration of how the media misinform the public about the issue, that same IOM review was reported by NPR under the headline "Schedule of Childhood Vaccines Declared Safe". Parents were told by NPR that the review "found there is no evidence that the federally recommended timeline for childhood vaccines is unsafe."[21]

What NPR withheld from the public is that this lack of evidence *arises from the fact that no studies have been done that are designed to examine the safety of the schedule by comparing health outcomes between children vaccinated according to the CDC's schedule and children who remain completely unvaccinated.*

What's more, government health officials have made it clear to parents that they should *not* expect such a study to be done.

The Institute of Medicine acknowledged in its 2013 review that the most informative study would be a randomized controlled trial comparing long-term health outcomes between children vaccinated according to the CDC's schedule and completely unvaccinated children. It nevertheless recommended that the government *not* initiate such a study on the grounds that it would be "unethical" to deprive children of the benefits of vaccines—the logical fallacy of begging the question.

The IOM instead recommended that the Department of Health and Human Services utilize an existing database called the Vaccine Safety Datalink (VSD), which is a collaborative project between the CDC and several health care organizations, to examine the safety of the CDC's schedule. It acknowledged that looking retrospectively at such data inherently risks selection biases that can invalidate findings. It also advised the government *against* dedicating a lot of funding to studying the schedule's safety on the grounds that it risked spending wastefully.[22]

By 2016, the CDC was still studying how to do a study examining long-term health outcomes to determine the safety of its routine childhood vaccine schedule.

In April 2016, the CDC published a white paper outlining its plans for following up on the IOM's recommendations. In it, the CDC stated that the IOM acknowledged that "few" studies had been done to examine the safety of the whole schedule, thus deceptively communicating that the number of such studies was more than *zero*.

Contradictorily, the CDC stated that a main purpose of the paper was to "Suggest methodological approaches that could be used to assess the safety of the recommended schedule as a whole"—thus tacitly acknowledging that this question about the safety of the schedule as a whole *had not yet been approached by researchers.*

The CDC also acknowledged that parents were demanding good data on how "child health outcomes compare between fully vaccinated and unvaccinated children" but suggested that such a study might not even be feasible using the VSD.

Instead, the CDC outlined a plan focused primarily on how a VSD study might be done comparing long-term health outcomes between children who were fully vaccinated and children who were also vaccinated, but not *strictly* in compliance with the CDC's schedule. It would be a "vaccination" versus "undervaccination" study of health outcomes for which a causal association with vaccines was biologically plausible.

Among these plausible outcomes were death; allergies and asthma; a broad range of autoimmune diseases, including irritable bowel diseases; circulatory system disorders; bone and joint diseases, including ankylosing spondylitis; demyelinating neurologic disorders; cardiovascular problems; seizures, including epilepsy; sudden infant death syndrome (SIDS); and a broad range of neurological system disorders including attention deficit disorder and autism.

The CDC acknowledged that among the problems of using the VSD to study the schedule's safety is the risk of "reverse causality". An example provided is of a parent who starts out vaccinating according to schedule but then observes early symptoms of a health problem they think is associated with the vaccinations and so chooses to delay or forego subsequent vaccines. While the CDC didn't explicitly acknowledge this as potential healthy vaccinee bias, the corollary is that this would result in children who are at greater risk being disproportionately represented in the "undervaccinated" cohort.

The CDC also explained that among the challenges of using the VSD to provide parents with a fully vaccinated versus fully unvaccinated study is the potential for misclassification. Just because a child has no record of vaccination in the database does not necessarily mean they were not vaccinated. Other records could be used to determine a negative vaccination history, but since the US childhood population is so highly vaccinated, the small number of unvaccinated children who could be included may be too small, leaving the study statistically underpowered.[23]

Meanwhile, public health officials across the country have been working hard to vaccinate away any potential unvaccinated cohort, including now in Oregon by delivering the clear message that pediatricians will risk losing their medical license if they insist on practicing informed consent.

Dr. Paul's Awakening

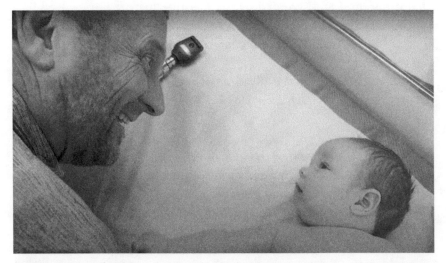

Dr. Paul Thomas works on getting a smile out of a two-month-old baby *(image from "A Crazy Day in the Life of a Busy Pediatrician" on Dr. Paul's YouTube channel).*[1]

In 1998, when Wakefield's paper was published in *The Lancet*, Dr. Paul Thomas was still doing what he had been *taught* to do: vaccinating children according to the CDC's recommendations. He had not yet joined the ranks of those whom he now broadly describes as "vaccine-risk aware."

"We all have our moments," Thomas explained. His own came when he read the paper by Andrew Wakefield. Prior to that, he had never seriously considered the possibility that vaccines could cause long-term harms to children.

"After reading it," Thomas related, "it just opened my mind to the fact that, 'Huh, maybe vaccines aren't all safe and effective,' right? So it was my first little wake-up call, and I owe that to Andy [Wakefield] because, you know, I didn't know anything, and I didn't wake up until I saw the one, two, three, four cases of autism that *totally* woke me up."

He was referring to his own experience as a pediatrician of witnessing young children regress into autism after vaccination, which compelled him onto "a journey to figure it out."

He began digging deeply into the medical literature. In 2003, he attended his first conference of a group called Defeat Autism Now! (DAN!), which was created under the Autism Research Institute. That program was disbanded by the institute in 2011 but evolved into another organization known as the Medical Academy of Pediatric Special Needs (MAPS), whose conferences on autism Thomas continued to attend.[2]

"Talk about deep, deep dive into science," Thomas said of the conferences, adding that AAP conferences were "weak" in their science by comparison.

The first case of regressive autism Thomas saw as a pediatrician was in 2004. He recalled having thought, "Oh, wow, so *that's* what that looks like." The next year, he saw a second case. Then yet another the following year. The fourth case came in November 2007.

"I remember it like it was yesterday, and I'm going to cry if I think too hard about it . . .," he said during our interview. After momentarily steeling himself, he continued: "Walked into a two-year-old visit, and he's supposed to be a well kid, and he's shaking his head back and forth and the lights are out of his eyes. There's nobody home. And mom was kind of in denial."

He said he was still taking care of that patient right up until the Oregon Medical Board suspended his license. "That was the last straw for me," Thomas continued. "I just couldn't go on with business as usual."

Thomas described what happened next with Westside Pediatrics as being "like a divorce". He approached his partners and expressed his concerns. They felt it was unethical to do anything other than what they were told by the CDC and AAP. Thomas felt it was unethical for him to continue the "standard of care" practice of treating vaccination as a one-size-fits-all solution to infectious disease.

As Thomas explained:

> I just ethically could no longer do business as usual, meaning the CDC's
> schedule, when I became very clearly aware of harm. We had harm from
> mercury—that was already out of the vaccines by 2008 except for the multi-
> dose flu shot; but also harm from aluminum. The data was overwhelming
> by that point with regards to how it was causing immune activation and
> direct toxicity. And then we also were starting to get information about
> immune activation as a way of creating autoimmunity, including attacking
> the brain. And just, you know, I mean an entire *book* on aluminum by
> Shoenfeld that showed the direct link with autoimmunity.

Autoimmune diseases are those in which the immune system is dysfunc-
tional, confusing self and non-self and attacking the body's own tissues
and organs as it would a foreign pathogenic invader.

The textbook Thomas was referring to is titled *Vaccines and
Autoimmunity*, the lead editor of which was Dr. Yehuda Shoenfeld, a
world-renowned Israeli scientist who heads a center for autoimmune
diseases at Sheba Medical Center in Tel Aviv and has published many
papers in top medical journals, including the *New England Journal of
Medicine*, *Nature*, and *The Lancet*. He is also on the editorial boards
of dozens of journals in the fields of rheumatology and autoimmunity
and is the founder and editor of the *Israel Medical Association Journal*
as well as of *Autoimmunity Reviews*. According to Sheba, he has published more than 1,750 papers. A search for papers on which he is listed
as an author in PubMed, an online database of peer-reviewed literature
operated by the National Institutes of Health, presently turns up 2,048
results.[3]

In 2008, after fifteen years with the group practice, Dr. Thomas left
Westside Pediatrics and opened his own clinic, Integrative Pediatrics, in
Beaverton. It was a move necessitated, he says, by his awakening to the
possibility that he was contributing to "iatrogenic" illness—meaning illness inadvertently caused by the well-intended interventions of medical
professionals.

Thomas was not alone in leaving the group practice. He says over
1,500 patients left with him, and the practice quickly grew to over 15,000,
with a staff of over thirty employees.

"And I went on my journey of, basically, honoring informed consent,"
Thomas said, describing this fundamental human right as "the one guid-
ing principle of Integrative Pediatrics".

Thomas said that none of the four cases of regressive autism he had witnessed involved sudden regression within just a few days of vaccination. He explained:

> I have those stories now. Lots of those stories in my practice. So, I have over one hundred severe autistic kids in my practice, and the stories are: they're at another pediatric office, and right after a vaccine or some time after a vaccine, they regress into severe autism. And the parents, you know, take their kids back to the pediatrician—what's really tragic, actually, sometimes they don't regress into full autism, but they're not quite right, and they come to the pediatrician and say, "You know, we're worried about these vaccines."
>
> And the pediatrician invariably says, "Oh, it's been proven, there's no link between vaccines and autism. Vaccines are safe and effective." They just spout off this, you know, marketing slogan as if it were a fact and *coerce* the patients into *continuing* to vaccinate an already vaccine-injured child. And they just keep pushing them further and further into a massive regression until finally they tip them into full-blown severe autism. I can't tell you how many times I've heard that story. Easily over a hundred times.
>
> And this is the thing: you know, if you're not a busy pediatrician who actually *listens* to the patients, and not actually having empathy and caring for those kinds of patients, and you're not listening to the fact that there's something going on—parents are *seeing* it, then you just *dismiss* those families. And, in fact, they often get discharged from my peers' practices for *not* following the CDC's schedule *despite* the fact that they're seeing damage in their kids.

While Dr. Thomas's clinic attracted parents of children who already had developed chronic health conditions or developmental disorders, he began noticing a marked difference in the health of patients whose parents were choosing *not* to follow the CDC's recommendations. "We started seeing that our less vaccinated or unvaccinated children seemed to be healthier," he said. "I mean it was palpable—you could just tell."

He had two waiting rooms in the practice: one for patients who were sick and another for those who were well. Over time, he says, fewer and fewer were coming into the sick waiting room. The pattern he describes over the past few years leading up to the suspension of his license by the

Oregon Medical Board is that of standing room only on the well side and an empty waiting room for sick patients.

This observation entrenched him further on the path that would ultimately prompt the Oregon Medical Board to take "emergency" action to stop him from caring for children as a licensed medical practitioner.

The fundamental difference that led to that confrontation is that Dr. Paul Thomas's primary goal is to achieve good health outcomes among his pediatric patients, whereas the overriding goal of the government is to achieve high vaccination rates.

As Thomas pursued his journey down the path of awakening and came to learn firsthand as a doctor how those goals directly conflicted with each other, he was confronted with a choice. He could shut up and stop asking questions, stop listening to the parents and instead dismiss their concerns, persuade himself that the unacceptably poor health of the childhood population had absolutely nothing to do with children receiving more than twenty vaccine doses by the time they reach their second year of age, and go on practicing pediatrics the way the bureaucrats expected him to; *or* he could act in the best interests of his patients *by standing up to the medical establishment.*

He had already expressed his decision by opening Integrative Pediatrics. But as he observed the pattern of superior health among children who received fewer or no vaccines, he was compelled to do more. It wasn't enough for him to help only those parents who had flocked to his clinic because he respected their right to make an informed choice about vaccination rather than pressuring them into compliance with the CDC's schedule. It wasn't enough to help only the children in his practice.

Just as when he faced the decision as a child of whether to step into line and raise the flag of an apartheid regime, Paul Thomas chose to do what he knew was right and accept the risk of being labeled a dangerous revolutionary. While he knew that he would be risking his career, he opted to essentially issue a very public challenge to the corrupt and abusive establishment.

Oregon State's Rejection of the Right to Informed Consent

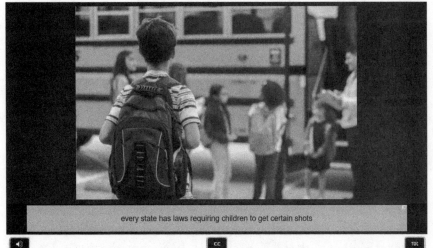

every state has laws requiring children to get certain shots

A screenshot from Oregon state government's "Vaccine Education Module," which contains misleading information about vaccines in pursuance of the policy goal of achieving high vaccine uptake *(accessible via Oregon.gov).*[1]

As Dr. Thomas continued his journey of awakening, the situation was becoming increasingly desperate for parents who viewed the "standard of care" with respect to vaccination as a threat to their children's health. As dissent increased, so did government policymakers' insistence on violating parents' right to informed consent.

The right to informed consent is one of the most fundamental ethics in medicine. The sole legitimate purpose of the government is to protect the rights of its citizens. Consequently, if we assume that legislators are acting in good faith within their authority derived from the consent of the governed, we should expect the right to informed consent to be enshrined in law.

And, indeed, Oregon law *requires* physicians "to obtain the informed consent of a patient", which means that doctors must inform patients of any "alternative procedures" and the risks involved in accepting a given treatment.

However, there is an aspect of this law that the Oregon Medical Board is now interpreting in bad faith and without authority. As the board appears to be interpreting this law, doctors are required to respect this right of patients *except* when it comes to vaccinations, in which case doctors are instead required to persuade or coerce patients into compliance rather than providing them with the knowledge required to make their own informed choice.

As the statute elaborates, if patients ask for more detailed information about a recommended medical intervention, physicians are required to "disclose in substantial detail the procedure, the viable alternatives and the material risks *unless to do so would be materially detrimental to the patient.*" (Emphasis added.)

In determining whether providing further explanation would be "detrimental", doctors must "give due consideration to the standards of practice" of "reasonable" medical practitioners "under the same or similar circumstances."[2]

The medical board seems to have interpreted this as meaning that pediatricians not only *can* but *must* persuade or coerce parents into vaccinating according to the CDC's schedule. In essence, the case of Dr. Paul Thomas illustrates how the board has assumed *a priori* that to do otherwise would be materially detrimental to children's health and, on that basis, concluded that physicians are therefore relieved of their legal and ethical responsibility to obtain fully informed consent.

Indeed, the message the Oregon Medical Board delivered to physicians by suspending Paul Thomas's license is that they will now be *required* to disregard and *violate* parents' right to informed consent. The pediatrician's job, as far as the state is concerned, is to support the policy goal of achieving high vaccination rates—which is fundamentally at odds with practicing informed consent.

The state government is simply not interested in answering any questions, whether from the parents or from the doctors, that challenge the dogma of their underlying assumption that for children *not* to comply with the CDC's schedule would be detrimental to their health.

In Oregon, parents are required to vaccinate their children according to the CDC's recommendations if they want their children to attend public school. This law fundamentally infringes on the right to informed consent because, rather than patients voluntarily *opting in* for vaccination, it places hurdles before them to opt *out*.

Until 2013, while the vaccine mandate was an infringement, parents still had options available to meaningfully exercise their right to not vaccinate. Children with conditions meeting the CDC's narrow range of criteria for recognized "contraindications" to vaccinations, such as having previously had a severe allergic reaction to a vaccine, could obtain a medical exemption from their doctor. Parents who had other reasons for opting out of one or more vaccines could sign a form to claim what is termed a "nonmedical" exemption (even if the reasons for declining vaccination are grounded in medical science).

That changed in 2013 with the passage of a law requiring parents to vault over a higher bar to obtain a "nonmedical" exemption. Now, parents would be required to receive what the state describes as "education" about the benefits and risks of "immunization" from either a health care professional or an "online vaccine education module" located on the website of the state's health department.

This mandated "education," however, was designed with a singular goal in mind: *to reduce the proportion of parents claiming nonmedical exemptions for their children.*[3]

The state simply wanted parents not to *choose* but *to obey*. Consequently, the so-called "education" was demonstrably intended *not* to inform but to *persuade* parents to vaccinate, which in turn necessitates *deceiving* them about the risks and benefits.

To judge the level of success toward attainment of the goal, the state would be measuring not child health outcomes but *vaccination rates*.

Government officials shroud their policies in the guise of "science," but *science simply does not tell us that poor health is caused by lack of vaccinations.*

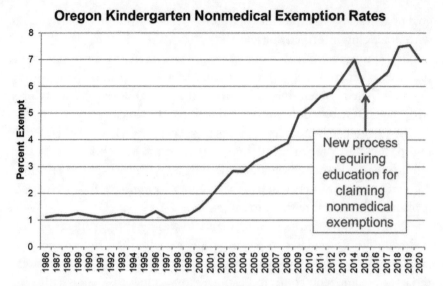

Oregon Kindergarten Nonmedical Exemption Rates

This graph from an Oregon Health Authority document illustrates the state's myopic focus on the goal of achieving high vaccination rates as opposed to the goal of achieving a healthy childhood population.[4]

Science does *not* tell us that humans evolved without a sufficiently functional immune system such that we all *require* pharmaceutical interventions *starting on the first day of our lives* to ensure good health. Science does *not* tell us that vaccines are a one-size-fits-all solution to infectious disease. Science does *not* tell us that if only *all* parents would strictly comply with the CDC's schedule, then we would not have such poor health among the childhood population.

What science and basic medical ethics are instead *screaming* at us is that *an individual risk-benefit analysis is required for the right to informed consent to be meaningfully exercised.* This analysis needs to be done for *each* vaccine *and each child.* Every vaccine has a different profile of safety and effectiveness. Not every child is at the same risk of the disease that a vaccine is intended to prevent. *Not every child is at the same risk of being harmed by the vaccine.*

What science is telling us is that without randomized placebo-controlled trials comparing long-term health outcomes, including all-cause mortality, between vaccinated and unvaccinated children, no meaningful claims about safety or effectiveness can be made.

What science tells us is that the statement that vaccines are "safe and effective" is an invalid generalization. After all, parents were told the same thing about the DTP and oral polio vaccines, yet they are no longer used in this country precisely because they came to be recognized as too risky even by public health officials. (Recall the FDA's attitude in 1984 that "any possible doubts, whether or not well founded, about the safety of the vaccine cannot be allowed to exist in view of the need to assure that the vaccine will continue to be used to the maximum extent consistent with the nation's public health objectives.")

The fact that some children are more susceptible to being harmed by vaccines has been acknowledged by the government, such as in a case decided in 2008 under the Vaccine Injury Compensation Program. At nineteen months of age, a girl named Hannah Poling, who had been developing normally, received nine vaccine doses at once. She developed a fever and encephalopathy and then developmentally regressed into diagnosed autism.

Hannah, whose father is a neurologist, happened to be a patient of an expert witness used by the government in VICP cases: Dr. Andrew Zimmerman, a pediatric neurologist, associate professor of neurology and psychiatry at the Johns Hopkins University School of Medicine, and director of medical research at the Kennedy Krieger Institute's Center for Autism and Related Disorders.

In one VICP case, the government's lawyers used Zimmerman's testimony to deny compensation to a child with autism. Dr. Zimmerman expressed his professional medical opinion that vaccines did not cause the patient's autism. As Zimmerman has since stated in an affidavit, he specifically told the government's lawyers that his opinion in that case was not generalizable to others.

Having witnessed what happened to young Hannah, Zimmerman told them that "in a subset of children with an underlying mitochondrial dysfunction, vaccine induced fever and immune stimulation that exceeded metabolic energy reserves could, and in at least one of my patients, did cause regressive encephalopathy with features of autism spectrum disorder."[5]

In a later case, the government's lawyers nevertheless proceeded to *deliberately misrepresent* Dr. Zimmerman's view by citing his opinion from the earlier case to deny compensation to another child with autism on the grounds that it was Zimmerman's view that vaccines do not cause autism. In fact, the conclusion Zimmerman arrived at for the latter case, after reviewing the child's medical records, was that he "suffered regressive encephalopathy with features of autism spectrum disorder as a result of a vaccine injury".[6]

In Hannah Poling's case, the government conceded that the vaccines she received "significantly aggravated an underlying mitochondrial disorder, which predisposed her to deficits in cellular energy metabolism, and manifested as a regressive encephalopathy with features of autism spectrum disorder."[7]

On March 29, 2008, CDC Director Julie Gerberding told the country on CNN, "Now, we all know that vaccines can occasionally cause fevers in kids. So, if a child was immunized, got a fever, had other complications from the vaccines, and if you're predisposed with a mitochondrial disorder, it can certainly set off some damage. Some of the symptoms can be symptoms that have characteristics of autism."[8]

Mitochondrial disorders are nevertheless *not* recognized by the CDC as a contraindication to vaccines that it recommends for routine use in children.

This is perhaps in part due to the difficulty of identifying such children. As the long-time director of the CDC's Immunization Safety Office, Dr. Frank DeStefano, acknowledged in an interview in 2018, "it's a possibility" that vaccines could cause autism in genetically susceptible individuals, but the problem is that it is "hard to predict who those children might be", and research designed to identify underlying cofactors that place certain children at greater risk of vaccine injury is "very difficult to do."[9]

That in turn helps to explain why the CDC doesn't do it. Instead, the government maintains its one-size-fits-all approach, treating those who are consequently harmed as lambs that must be laid on the sacrificial altar in the name of "public health" while the high priests of the vaccine religion go on proclaiming the dogma that vaccines are "safe and effective."

It is a simple logical truism that government bureaucrats *do not have the requisite knowledge of the individual child* to be able to conduct a *meaningful* risk-benefit analysis on that child's behalf. *Only the child's parents or legal guardians, in consultation perhaps with the child's pediatrician, have that essential knowledge.*

The bureaucrats nevertheless arrogantly proclaim to know better. This brings us back to the "education" that parents in Oregon are required to receive before they are permitted an exemption for what they *mistakenly* call "nonmedical" exemptions no matter how firmly the parental choice is grounded in medical science.

On the "Nonmedical Vaccine Exemptions" page of the Oregon state government's website, Oregon.gov, one can view the "Vaccine Education Module" parents are expected to sit through to obtain a "nonmedical" exemption, if they prefer that route, or if their child's pediatrician simply will not sign an exemption for them—such as parents who are expelled from a practice for declining vaccinations.

The introduction video states that "parents should have science-based information before claiming an exemption". Certainly, it is true that parents must have science-based information to be able to make an informed choice, but while the module purports to provide that, even a cursory examination of its contents reveals that it is propaganda, not educational material.

Notably, parents who *do* comply with the state's demands to vaccinate their children according to the CDC's schedule are not required to receive the same "education" about the risks and benefits of doing so, which is itself sufficient to demonstrate that the goal here is *not* to obtain informed consent but to *prevent* informed consent from happening.

An immediate example of unscientific information is how the introduction video equates "immunity" with "antibodies" as measured in the blood.[10] In truth, a high level of antibodies is neither always sufficient nor even necessary for immunity. There are also mechanisms of innate and cellular immunity that are importantly involved—and the narrow focus on antibodies with vaccination is an illustration of the institutional myopia that exists within the medical establishment.

One of the reasons this misleading information is so significant is that parents are *wrongly* taught to believe that vaccines confer the exact same type of immunity as infection, but without the individual having to experience disease symptoms. When this suggestion is made, all they are really saying is that both infection and vaccination stimulate the production of antibodies. All the *differences* in immune responses are completely ignored.

Hence, *opportunity costs* related to vaccination are also completely ignored.

As an example of opportunity cost, the immunity conferred by the acellular pertussis vaccine (DTaP) differs from that conferred by the older whole-cell vaccine (DTP). Because the latter included the whole organism and not selected antigen components only, the immunity it conferred more closely resembled that conferred by infection. For example, infection confers not only a robust humoral, or antibody, response, but also mucosal immunity, which is important for preventing infection in the lungs.

Due to mechanisms related to the *inferiority* of the immunity conferred by the pertussis vaccine, "all children who were primed by DTaP vaccines", as opposed to natural infection or the whole-cell vaccine, "will be more susceptible to pertussis throughout their lifetimes, and there is no easy way to decrease this increased lifetime susceptibility." That was the conclusion of a review published in the *Journal of the Pediatric Infectious Diseases Society* in 2019.[11]

Another consequence is that the pertussis vaccine *does not prevent transmission*, thus resulting in a greater proportion of asymptomatic carriers who may pose an even *greater* risk to infant siblings who are too young to get vaccinated because, had the older child experienced symptoms, the family would have known to keep the siblings apart until resolution.[12]

There are, of course, numerous other important examples of opportunity costs, but they would be superfluous for our purposes here to mention. The point is that one would *think* that this type of information would be valuable to parents *and indeed necessary* for them to be able to make a truly *informed* choice. But, of course, the state does not *want* them to choose; it wants them to *obey*. Hence the mistakenly simplistic equation of "antibodies" with "immunity" in Oregon state's "education" module.

And, naturally, many parents who choose not to strictly comply with the CDC's schedule *already know these things because they've done their own research*, which is why forcing them to endure this so-called "education" serves only to insult their intelligence.

The video goes on to state that vaccines confer herd immunity, which is needed to protect those who can't get vaccinated, thus misleading parents into the mistaken belief that, for example, if they get their older child the pertussis vaccine, it will stop the child from transmitting the virus to the newborn baby. This is the *opposite* of informed consent.

The introduction video also misleads parents about the adequacy of the safety studies that have been done. It presents the argument that we can trust that vaccines are safe because they require FDA approval and a recommendation by the CDC's advisory committee to be added to the schedule, but this, too, simply insults parents' intelligence, the first fallacy being the false premise that these agencies are trustworthy and the second being the non sequitur that *if* a vaccine goes through these processes, *therefore* it is safe.

It goes further by adding that, for each vaccine, the CDC considers "whether it can be given at the same time as other vaccines." That statement may be literally true. We may reasonably suppose that they "consider" it. But what matters isn't whether they've "considered" it, but whether they've adequately studied it. This statement is transparently intended to lead parents to the conclusion that studies have been done showing that it's safe for them to vaccinate according to the CDC's schedule when, as observed by the Institute of Medicine, that is untrue.[13]

In this context, the video presents the deputy health officer for Multnomah County, "Dr. Vines," discussing how she vaccinated her own child due to her strong *faith* in the safety of adhering to the CDC's schedule: "I had no doubts about giving several vaccines at the same time because kids' immune systems can easily handle them. There's excellent science supporting the safety of vaccines."

This person's *belief* in vaccine safety and her *opinion* that the quality of studies and regulatory standards of evidence supporting the safety of the CDC's schedule is "excellent" tell us *precisely nothing* about the science. The only thing this segment of the video is evidence for *is that many public health officials believe their own propaganda.*

Of course, public health officials have already lost that argument: as we've already seen, the federal government has *conceded* that some children, such as those with a mitochondrial disorder, may *not* be able to handle numerous vaccines administered at once. Once again, the "education" module serves only to insult the intelligence of parents who do their own research and who perhaps should be the ones teaching public health officials about vaccine science.

There are numerous additional examples of how state health officials are *misinforming* parents just from the introduction video, but the point is sufficiently illustrated: *the state's "Vaccine Education Module" is*

*not intended to help parents make an informed choice but to deceive them
into compliance so that willfully ignorant and authoritarian policymakers can
achieve their myopic goal of high vaccination rates.*

It's not difficult to understand, then, why parents who do *not* consent
to the state's vaccine mandate and do *not* wish to suffer the humiliation
of being so insulted by arrogant and hypocritical government officials end
up taking their children to see "Dr. Paul."

Punishing Doctors for Serving Their Patients Rather Than the State

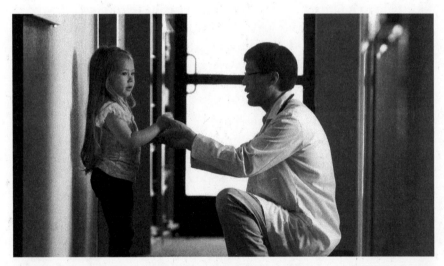

Senator Richard Pan, a practicing pediatrician, has led the California state government's efforts to systematically violate parents' right to informed consent for vaccinations *(photo by Dr. Richard Pan, licensed under CC BY-SA 2.0).*[1]

Paul Thomas's approach of grounding his practice in the principle of *informed consent* and focusing on *health outcomes* stands in stark contrast to the approach taken by the state government of violating informed consent to achieve high vaccination rates.

Oregon, of course, is not alone. *All* the states have taken the approach of mandating vaccinations for school attendance. In the extremity of its coercion, Oregon was outdone by California, which in 2016 passed a law *eliminating* "nonmedical" exemptions.

However, that did not have the intended effect because it incentivized parents to go to pediatricians who are respectful of informed consent to obtain a medical exemption. The problem, as perceived by those myopically focused on achieving high vaccination rates, was that physicians might grant exemptions "for indications outside of accepted contraindications", such as on the basis of "family medical history".[2]

The law was considered to "work" based on whether it increased the childhood vaccination rate rather than on whether it achieved a healthier childhood population. Pediatricians who would write medical exemptions for reasons such as the patient having a family history of autoimmune disease were regarded as "accomplices"—as though by enabling parents to exercise their right to informed consent they were engaging in *criminal* activity.[3]

The state senator who spearheaded the elimination of "nonmedical" exemptions, Dr. Richard Pan, subsequently introduced a bill he described as being intended to strengthen "oversight" of physicians to stop them from writing "fake" medical exemptions, which were those found by the state "to be fraudulent *or inconsistent with contraindications to vaccination per CDC guidelines*."[4] (Emphasis added.)

With the passage of that bill into law in September 2019, the state declared for itself the authority to *revoke* medical exemptions written by licensed physicians, with the clear warning communicated to doctors that if they write exemptions for any reasons other than CDC-defined contraindications, the state was going to come after them for their "unscrupulous" behavior.[5]

Richard Pan expressed his view on the matter very clearly in a commentary in the AAP's journal *Pediatrics*. When physicians write medical exemptions to state vaccine mandates, he wrote, it is "not the practice of medicine but of a state authority to licensed physicians" who are "fulfilling an administrative role" on behalf of the state.[6]

Thus, in Pan's view, the state's proper role is to insert itself into the doctor-patient relationship by dictating how pediatricians should practice medicine, *and informed consent for the parents is not an option.*

Incidentally, according to the *Sacramento Bee*, California legislators had received $2 million from pharmaceutical companies, with Richard

Pan having received $95,000, in the two years prior to the passage of the first bill eliminating nonmedical exemptions.[7]

The message delivered by the second law was underscored by the state's prior treatment of Dr. Bob Sears, who published a book in 2007 titled *The Vaccine Book* in response to growing parental concerns about the safety of vaccinating their children according to the CDC's schedule. In the book, Dr. Sears provided an alternative schedule to allay concerns and to guide parents who wish to do fewer vaccines or to space them out more.[8]

Among the sins committed by Sears in his book were informing parents that doctors like him learn very little about vaccines in medical school and should listen to and be open to learning from parents who've done more research, acknowledging that the CDC and pharmaceutical industry are untrustworthy, advocating respect for the right to informed consent, failing to instill proper fear into parents of the diseases for which there are vaccines, and informing parents that there are important differences in the immunity conferred by vaccines versus infection.[9]

In 2016, the California Medical Board charged Dr. Sears with "professional misconduct" and threatened to revoke his license for having enabled a mother to exercise her right to decline further vaccinations for her two-year-old child by writing a letter exempting her from all future vaccinations. In the state's judgment, the fact that the mom was concerned because the boy had gone "limp 'like a ragdoll' lasting 24 hours" and was "not himself for up to a week" after receiving his three-month-old vaccines was insufficient reason for Sears to write the exemption.

Incidentally, that charge was leveled at Sears by Kamala D. Harris, the current vice president of the United States, who was then attorney general of California.[10]

The result was that in 2018, Dr. Sears was placed under a thirty-five-month probation for "deviating from standards of care" by respecting the mother's right to decline further vaccinations on the *medical* grounds that the boy had previously suffered a serious reaction that would no doubt cause *any* parent to think twice *and avoid the risk of doing the same thing again to their child.*

Dr. Pan's coauthor on his *Pediatrics* paper expressing his authoritarian view on the practice of medicine, UC Hastings law professor Dorit Reiss, described the exemption written by Dr. Sears as "unjustified".[11] The *Los Angeles Times* accurately explained that Dr. Sears' sin was having written "a doctor's note for a 2-year-old boy exempting him from all childhood vaccinations." The case was settled when he stipulated that he had done so because of the mother's reasonable concern.[12]

As the authors of an article in *Pediatrics* understatedly remarked, the punishment meted out to Sears for practicing informed consent "may be a signal to other physicians who write medical exemptions outside the intent of the law that they may face similar consequences."[13]

That message was made all the louder and clearer by the passage of the law in 2019 putting physicians on notice that if they grant medical exemptions for reasons unapproved by the bureaucrats, they will face similar punishment.

Dr. Paul's Vaccine-Friendly Plan

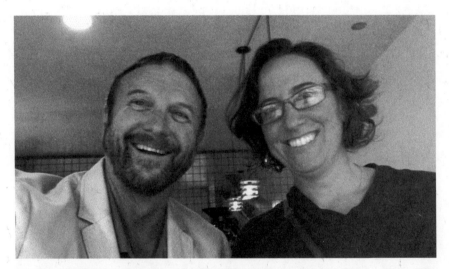

Dr. Paul Thomas and Dr. Jennifer Margulis, authors of the book *The Vaccine-Friendly Plan (photo courtesy of Paul Thomas)*

In 2015, the year before California's government took the step of eliminating nonmedical exemptions, Dr. Paul Thomas saw the writing on the wall in terms of the politics surrounding the practice of vaccination and commissioned a quality assurance analysis of his patients' data.

As he explained, what he had been seeing in his practice was that the children of parents who were choosing *not* to comply with the CDC's schedule were coming in to see him for chronic health conditions less frequently or not at all. It was difficult for him to escape the conclusion that his unvaccinated patients were *healthier* than those who were vaccinated. This included incidences of autism.

"People misquote me and say that I'm saying, 'Vaccines cause autism,'" Thomas said. "No, that's not what I'm saying. I'm saying I was *observing* vaccinated children regressing into autism at a *much* higher rate than the unvaccinated."

But it wasn't just autism. He said, "I was seeing a reduction in my unvaccinated kids of nearly all chronic disease."

Thomas said that the data from the 2015 quality assurance analysis confirmed his empirical observations. He considered getting approval from the state's Institutional Review Board to publish the findings, but he ended up never pursuing publication of the deidentified data. "That's on me," he said, expressing regret about not having done so at the time. It was a considerable undertaking and not his personal skill set.

However, what he saw in the data *did* prompt him to take a step he had thought about previously, which was to write a book on the subject. He had previously figured that Dr. Sears's book was already out there to help parents navigate the conflicting information and make the choice that was right for their children, so there was no need to undertake that effort. However, what he saw from his own patients' data compelled him to write a book of his own: *The Vaccine-Friendly Plan.*

His purpose, he explained, was to help parents understand the whole issue "and the importance of individualizing how you think about vaccines, that we really shouldn't have a one-size-fits-all schedule."

The "plan" was not so much a single rigidly regimented alternative to the CDC's schedule but the simple concept that parents should decide for themselves whether and when to vaccinate their children. His aim was to provide parents with the information they would need to be able to make their own informed choice. The book, coauthored with Dr. Jennifer Margulis, was published in August 2016.

Dr. Thomas knew then that he was risking his career by taking that step. Referring to the medical board's suspension of his license, he says that he knew that this day had been coming from the moment his book was published.

He said he knew he was risking his career because *The Vaccine-Friendly Plan* "takes on the CDC's schedule," and "the CDC's schedule is sacred."

When asked whether he recalled ever seeing regressive autism in *unvaccinated* children in his practice, Thomas promptly answered, "Yes. I have one."

That segued Thomas into a discussion about how the first chapter of his book is on environmental toxins. There are *many* factors in the development of autism, he explains, and the exposures children receive from the CDC's vaccine schedule must be understood as *additive* to their toxic burden from countless other sources.

To provide an illustration of his point, when the FDA acknowledged in 2001 that the levels of mercury to which infants were being exposed exceeded the government's own safety guidelines, it was considering *only* the amount of mercury children received from vaccines, *without* considering synergistic toxicity with aluminum adjuvants concomitantly administered *or* the toxic burden they were already carrying from other environmental exposures.

There are also genetic vulnerabilities that must be considered, Thomas added. This brought him back to autism, which he thinks is "not really a helpful label."

What he means is that the term is used to describe a broad array of developmental and behavioral abnormalities for which the medical establishment has no clear explanation. Indeed, this is reflected by the official diagnostic name itself: "autism spectrum disorder," or "ASD."

At that point, Thomas came back to the question about whether he had any unvaccinated children with autism in his practice, adding that the mother of the one case, to the best of his knowledge, had also not received any vaccines during pregnancy.

This raises a whole other issue apart from the risk of vaccinating young children. The effects on the developing fetus from vaccinating pregnant women are a big unknown. We're supposed to believe otherwise. We're told that it's "safe." But this claim rests on such a flimsy scientific basis that the CDC's safety claim is directly contradicted by what the vaccine manufacturers themselves disclose about it in their package inserts.

The CDC recommends the flu shot for pregnant women, proclaiming that this practice is "safe" despite flu shots being classified by the FDA as pharmaceutical products for which there are either "no adequate and well-controlled studies in pregnant women" or "no adequate and well-controlled studies in humans".

As a review published in the *American Journal of Obstetrics & Gynecology* in 2012 observed, "prelicensure data on influenza vaccine safety and effectiveness during pregnancy is virtually nonexistent", and "data from observational studies do not reach the standard" set by the FDA for assessing safety. Hence, the FDA's classification of flu shots "is indicative of a lack of available data to demonstrate vaccine safety in pregnancy".[1]

The reason prelicensure data on the safety of vaccination during pregnancy are virtually nonexistent is that pregnant women *are excluded* from clinical trials on the grounds that to subject them to experimentation would be unethical.

This raises an obvious question: If it is considered unethical to include pregnant women in clinical trials, how is it not *also* unethical to recommend that all pregnant women be vaccinated in the *absence* of randomized, placebo-controlled studies demonstrating this to be safe? In what way does the CDC's flu shot recommendation *not* treat a pregnant woman and the child developing in her womb *as subjects of a mass uncontrolled experiment without their informed consent?*

Indeed, were the vaccine manufacturers themselves to make the same claims about the safety of vaccinating pregnant women as the CDC, *they could be sued for fraud.* That's *precisely* why they state *right in their package inserts* that the safety and effectiveness of their products "have not been established in pregnant women or nursing mothers."[2]

Coming back to the conversation with Thomas, he did express one regret about his decision to publish the book: "I realized after writing *The Vaccine-Friendly Plan*," he lamented, "that it wasn't friendly enough."

The Oregon Medical Board Takes Aim at Dr. Paul

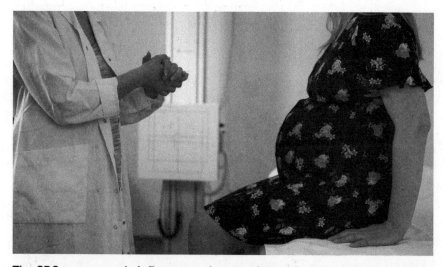

The CDC recommends influenza and pertussis vaccines for pregnant women despite the vaccine manufacturers stating in their package inserts that adequate safety studies have not been done to determine the risk of this practice *(public domain photo courtesy of Max Pixel)*.[1]

The first accusation from the Oregon Medical Board came on December 26, 2018. Thomas received a letter of complaint describing what he says was an unsubstantiated allegation. He was accused of having provided care related to vaccinations during pregnancy and early childhood that was "not consistent with the CDC, American Academy of Pediatrics, and other evidence based medicine practices."[2]

"They gave us the name," Thomas said, "so we were able to track the name, and they're not in our practice. So there's no evidence that this was actually a person who came into my practice."

Thomas's attorney notified the Oregon Medical Board in a letter dated January 11, 2019, that the child identified in the letter as being the subject of the complaint "was apparently never a patient of Dr. Thomas, nor any of the care providers in his clinic."[3]

"Regardless," Thomas explained, "the vaccines for pregnancy on the package insert say very specifically 'not tested for pregnancy.' So the CDC is making a recommendation that is experimenting on pregnant women in America, and that goes on to this day. And they want that to continue because, well, clearly, they're going after my license, and the first complaint was over *that* issue."

Indeed, as noted, flu shot manufacturers state right in their product package inserts that adequate safety studies have not been done to determine the risk of what amounts to *deliberately* causing an *inflammatory* response during pregnancy.

For example, GlaxoSmithKline's flu shot product Fluarix states that the "[s]afety and effectiveness of FLUARIX while pregnant have not been established in pregnant women or nursing mothers." There are "no adequate and well-controlled studies in pregnant women."[4] Sanofi Pasteur's Fluzone insert likewise states that "Safety and effectiveness of Fluzone has not been established in pregnant women." It is "not known whether Fluzone can cause fetal harm when administered to a pregnant woman or can affect reproduction capacity."[5] Seqirus's Fluvirin insert states, "Safety and effectiveness of FLUVIRIN® have not been established in pregnant women" or "nursing mothers". There are "no adequate and well-controlled studies in pregnant women."[6]

Inflammation during pregnancy is *known* to cause "abnormalities in brain development associated with subsequent cognitive impairment and an increased susceptibility to schizophrenia and autism spectrum disorders." A study published in *Nature* in December 2020 notes that maternal immune activation therefore "may contribute to the underlying pathophysiological mechanisms linking maternal immune status to subsequent risks for cognitive disease."[7]

Additionally, multidose vials of influenza vaccine contain ethylmercury, which can be transported through the placental barrier as well as into the brain, where it breaks down into inorganic mercury and accumulates.

As noted in one of the studies that the CDC cites to support its claim that the mercury in flu shots is "safe," inorganic mercury in the brain has been "associated with a significant increase in the number of microglia in the brain", and "'an active neuroinflammatory process' has been demonstrated in brains of autistic patients, including a marked activation of microglia."[8]

The CDC also recommends the aluminum-containing tetanus, diphtheria, and pertussis (Tdap) vaccine for pregnant women, whereas, once again, the manufacturers state that adequate studies have not been done to determine the safety of this practice. Sanofi's Adacel insert states, "There are no adequate and well-controlled studies of Adacel administration in pregnant women in the U.S."[9] GlaxoSmithKline's product similarly states, "There are no adequate and well-controlled studies of BOOSTRIX in pregnant women in the U.S."[10]

Dr. Thomas said that what likely happened in this case, assuming it was a real complaint, was that, in addition to informing the expectant mother of the CDC's recommendation, he went over the disclosures contained in the manufacturer's package insert with the woman, which is something most other doctors would likely not have done.

In other words, the board had essentially accused him of having practiced informed consent.

Thomas added that, around the time he received that complaint, he also got a call from a doctor who warned that his wife was involved in a private Facebook group for physician spouses whose members planned to target Thomas with repeated board complaints.

Multiple additional complaints came in 2019. Thomas described these also as being unsubstantiated, with none of the complaints appearing to have come from any of his actual patients.

In its December 2018 letter of complaint, the Oregon Medical Board requested Dr. Thomas to explain why his vaccine-friendly plan differs from the CDC schedule and to "[p]rovide any published peer reviewed medical journal articles that supports your vaccination schedule."[11]

This request prompted Thomas to hire an independent pediatrician and informatics expert to do a quality assurance project looking at health outcomes of all patients born into his practice.

That was an important inclusion criterion. As Thomas explained, "Most of the patients who come to our practice, or at least a very significant percentage of them, come because they have health problems that they are worried were triggered by vaccines, and they can't get their pediatrician, wherever they are, to slow down or stop vaccinating, and so they come to the only safe place they can find."

This meant that he was "getting a lot of damaged kids already," whereas "very, very few" of those born into his practice had comparable health problems.

To include children who came to him from other practices would introduce a confounding factor that would bias the results. What he wanted to know was what kind of outcomes were resulting from various numbers of vaccinations received among patients who *from the start* were with a clinic *that practices informed consent.*

The board's request that Thomas provide evidence to support "the vaccine-friendly plan" *ignored* the fact that *the CDC's schedule has not been scientifically demonstrated to be safer than not vaccinating at all*, as tacitly acknowledged by the Institute of Medicine.[12] It's just "standard of care."

The board's request also illustrates how government policymakers *do not even understand how informed consent works.*

"I don't 'do' the vaccine-friendly plan," Thomas explained. "We simply do informed consent." Yes, the book presents one way of doing it, he said, "but I don't push it." To do that would be contrary to the whole idea of individualized care.

There is a "really important" caveat to that, he added. "We have the approach of, when we see developmental delays or child development stalling out, we stop. We don't keep pushing the vaccine schedule. We offer to the parents the concept that, 'Perhaps vaccines are triggering this delay that we're seeing, so why don't we hold off and just see how your child does between now and your next well-child visit.'"

Parents who follow the vaccine-friendly plan specifically according to the book "are probably the most vaccinated in this dataset," he noted. Parents rarely want more vaccination than that. After pausing momentarily to think about it, he added that it amounts to roughly half the doses of the CDC's schedule.

There is an important point to be made here. Given what studies show about the problem of "healthy vaccinee" bias in observational studies, we should expect that children *predisposed* to certain health conditions would be *more* likely pooled into the unvaccinated group.

One reason for this is that parents avoid vaccines for younger siblings if the older siblings experienced vaccine-related adverse events, as already discussed. Another is that, regardless of birth order, parents of children who start showing symptoms earlier in life may be more likely to avoid subsequent vaccinations.

Consequently, there may be an inherent bias in his data *against* the hypothesis that vaccinating less is associated with better health outcomes.

When this possibility was raised with him, he responded, "There is no question that I carry a much higher burden of high-risk families because I get a lot of the patients who had one autistic child or maybe two, they finally wake up to what's going on; they say, we're not vaccinating our next kid, and then those kids get enrolled into the study—because they were born into the practice."

Thinking about it a moment further, he reiterated, "Right. You would expect to find more illness and more disease incidence in my unvaccinated because they're at higher risk—and despite that variable, which is very real, we still have robust findings."

He was referring to the findings published in a peer-reviewed journal just days before the medical board issued an "emergency" suspension of his license.

Coming back to how he practices informed consent, Thomas talked about how, with motor skills such as learning how to walk, there is a "big bell curve" in terms of variability. But, socially, if a child is not making eye contact by four to six months of age, that is a big red flag.

"I'm a nut," he said. "If I can't get a smile, there's something wrong."

He described a phenomenon of "gaze aversion" with some babies, which is "a clue." Elaborating on what he would say to the parents in such a situation, he continued:

> "If I were in your shoes—here's the CDC schedule, here's what's recommended. If it were my baby—I'm not telling you what to do." This is nuance of informed consent that is I think important. I think physicians should not tell people what to do, but they *should* be honest and tell them what *they* would do if they were in that person's shoes.
>
> I mean, most patients want to know that because—I think because of the legalities of what's going on in the world today, they say, "This is the CDC's schedule. This is what we want you to do."
>
> "If I were in your shoes, would you want to know what I would do?" I actually ask them before I tell them, and they almost always say, "Of course I want to know!" And so I tell them. So I'm not telling them what to do; I'm

telling them what *I* would do. "I would slow down and make sure we're not tipping that child over the edge. I've seen it happen too many times where kids get tipped over the edge."

He also commented further on the one regret he has with his book:

> I would propose that *The Vaccine-Friendly Plan* is a compromise. It's not ideal, but it's certainly better than the CDC schedule as far as the amount of harm it's going to cause. I mean, that's just an extrapolation. We can't really say that from this data. So, to look at the harm from the CDC schedule, you just have to look at population rates. What's the current population rate for autism, for ADHD, for asthma, for eczema? That data is out there. So, then you take that data, and you compare it to my data, and you go, "Oh, okay, well, it sure appears that following the vaccine-friendly plan, or some version of it, is *very* beneficial for health outcomes."

For example, his published data show that *none* of his unvaccinated patients had attention deficit hyperactivity disorder (ADHD), compared to 5.3 percent of patients who had been vaccinated to one extent or another. The 5.3 percent of variably vaccinated patients with ADHD further compares with the national rate, according to the CDC, of 9.3 percent.[13]

Asked to comment on this, Thomas responded, "I don't know. That just blows my mind, actually, that that's what we found."

There were too few children with autism in Thomas's practice to include in the published statistical analysis, but the rate in his clinic can still be compared with the rate among the general childhood population. Among patients born into his practice, 0.36 percent had autism. The national rate for ASD, according to the CDC, is 1.85 percent.

Therefore, without insinuating anything about causality, we can fairly say that being born into Dr. Paul's practice is associated with a fivefold *decreased* risk of being diagnosed with autism compared to the general population of *highly vaccinated* children.[14]

Pressed further to explain why there were so few ADHD and autism patients in his practice when, according to the CDC's prevalence estimates, we should expect there to be considerably more, Thomas replied, "What really saves them is you have to be very observant at every well-child visit, and you stop vaccinating if you see any problems."

Putting himself again in the shoes of parents who had come to him from other practices, he added, "Many doctors will say, 'Oh that's normal.' *No!* It's 'normal' *today* for *most* pediatricians because they see it all the time. It's the 'new normal.' But that is *not* normal."[15]

Having been asked by the Oregon Medical Board to produce evidence that following his vaccine-friendly plan results in equal or better health outcomes as does following the CDC's schedule, Thomas commissioned the quality assurance project. However, he approached it a bit unconventionally. He did it to look at *health outcomes*, he stressed, not "how well you can follow a protocol."

Most "quality assurance" projects looking at vaccines, he explained, are looking at whether physicians did them or not. "That doesn't reflect on the health of what those vaccines are doing one iota."

The scientist he commissioned to analyze his data, Thomas said, initially expressed his skepticism that his unvaccinated kids were really doing so much better than others. But by the end of the first day of going over the data, the analyst said, "Paul, this is unbelievable! The data literally jumps out at you."

"Right, so what he was seeing," Thomas continued, "was massive increases in health problems in the highly vaccinated and a massive decrease in health problems in the unvaccinated. And it was undeniable."

He came back to the fundamental question that the state medical board was really asking of him: "Is the process of allowing patients informed consent—is that causing harm?" Expressing justified frustration, he continued:

> Because what's happening in most other practices: parents are handed a two-page "vaccine information statement" [from the CDC], which is very uninformative, and they're told, "Here's your information about the vaccine. The nurse will be in to give you your shot." *That's* "informed consent" in most offices today. It's *nothing*. It's *no* information.
>
> It's an assumption—*presumption*—that you're going to do the shots. *All* of them. And end of story. No questions. They actually *train* pediatricians in how to avoid taking questions. So informed consent is *not* going on *except* in a few practices around the country like mine where we actually make the effort to do the process.

Dr. Thomas had already demonstrated a willingness to question his core beliefs when he departed from his training in the first place so that he could start practicing informed consent. Now that he was under fire for straying from "standard of care," that willingness to be self-critical continued to present itself.

"Am I actually causing harm?" Thomas asked himself, this time in the context of his decision to leave the group practice and open Integrative Pediatrics. "Because if I am, I need to know that. So, it's the most ethical thing you can do—look actually at your data."

After commissioning the quality analysis project, Dr. Thomas got the approval of the state's institutional review board to publish the deidentified data. Working together with research scientist Dr. James Lyons-Weiler, also known as Dr. Jack, he analyzed and published his data in November 2020.

In the meantime, the attacks on Dr. Thomas continued. An article written by Rachel Monahan and published on the Portland-based news website *Willamette Week* on March 20, 2019, illustrates the lack of seriousness with which the news media approach the topic of public vaccine policy.

A Local Newspaper Joins in the Attacks on Dr. Paul

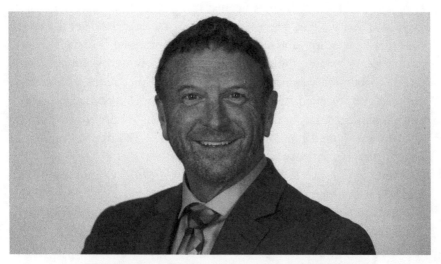

Dr. Paul Thomas, MD *(photo courtesy of Paul Thomas)*

In the *Willamette Week* article, Dr. Thomas was described as "Oregon's leading dissenter from scientific consensus." His book *The Vaccine-Friendly Plan* is an "anti-vaxx bible." He "hawks vitamins and supplements" and tells parents "that their suspicion vaccines cause autism is true."[1]

The key accusation in the article is that Thomas was misinforming parents and bullying them into *not* vaccinating their children, engaging in "unsubstantiated fear-mongering and internet conspiracy theories", and irresponsibly scaring parents with the "scientifically disproven" claim that vaccines cause autism.

To support this characterization of Dr. Thomas, Monahan cited a Michigan physician named David Gorski, whom she described as "managing editor of Science-Based Medicine, a journal that works to dispel misinformation about medical science". Gorski described Thomas as "a rising star in the anti-vaccine movement" who "should know better" than to "claim that children today are not as healthy as they were in the past."[2]

Next, the article presented another Portland pediatrician named Dr. Jay Rosenbloom, who is associated with a group called Boost Oregon "that is dedicated to vaccine education". Rosenbloom "says he regularly sees parents who previously went to Thomas." Parents go to Thomas to protect their children with vaccinations, Rosenbloom was quoted as saying, but Thomas "tries to pressure them out of it".[3]

Then the article shifted into presenting a glimpse of Dr. Thomas's side of the story, explaining how he opened Integrative Pediatrics after observing four of his patients regress into autism. He explained to *Willamette Week* that he was not "anti-vaccine" but "pro-informed consent."

In Oregon's state capital, Salem, the article reported, lawmakers were "trying to eliminate nonmedical exemptions", but "outraged mothers" protested the proposed legislation, reflecting how Oregon had become "a national battleground for the anti-vaxx movement." A mom at the protest in Salem was quoted expressing a positive view of Thomas, saying that he "really values his patients' opinion".

Although Thomas had told Monahan that he fully vaccinated his own children, recommends vaccines in his book, vaccinates children in his practice, and was not anti-vaccine, *Willamette Week* described him as the "king" of the "anti-vaxx movement".

The remainder of the article was dedicated to portraying Thomas as a doctor who rejected science by propagating "the vaccination-autism" myth and who ran a practice that had lower vaccination rates because he bullied parents into signing refusal forms.

Monahan recounted the story of a six-year-old unvaccinated boy who was hospitalized for tetanus in 2017. "When he left the hospital, he once again did not receive the vaccine," she reported. "The pediatrician that consulted with the family and signed his discharge papers? Dr. Paul Thomas."

"Thomas says the family called him but declines to say more, citing patient confidentiality," Monahan added.

Finally, *Willamette Week* presented the story of Leah Klass, a forty-two-year-old mom who said she had taken her second daughter in to see Thomas for her first vaccinations, but that he instead told her to sign a form saying she wanted to decline the vaccines. "He says wouldn't I feel terrible as a mother," Klass was quoted as saying, "if my child later developed autism and wouldn't I feel terrible if I could have prevented it?"[4]

The article then quoted Thomas denying the incident, but this was presented in parentheses, as though the fact that he denied that it ever happened were not directly pertinent to the accusation.

Klass further accused Thomas of "manipulating" parents into not vaccinating their children and "actively prohibiting a normal vaccine schedule". The article also relayed that "Klass thinks the Oregon Medical Board should investigate Thomas." Gorski was also further quoted agreeing that state medical boards should discipline "anti-vaccine doctors" who do not practice "according to the standard of care" by ensuring that their patients are vaccinated strictly according to the CDC's schedule.

The conclusion the public was left with by the *Willamette Week* article was that Thomas was a "menace" to society who should be "stripped of his license."[5]

On the webpage where it elicits donations for its journalism fund, *Willamette Week* describes Monahan's article as "[a] chilling profile of a prominent physician and best-selling author who believes that measles vaccinations may cause Autism. At a moment when the Northwest is suffering a measles epidemic, Dr. Paul Thomas is giving cover to thousands of Oregon parents who choose to avoid vaccines, thus jeopardizing the rest of Oregon's youth."[6]

Contrary to this reporting, Dr. Thomas says that during the measles outbreak he was able to give hundreds of MMR vaccines to patients who had previously refused these vaccines. It was precisely because he honors informed consent that these families trusted him and were willing to get the vaccine when measles was in the community. None of his patients came down with measles.

The *Willamette Week* article provided no credible evidence that Dr. Thomas was guilty of any wrongdoing. On the contrary, it is a perfect illustration of how the media are generally incompetent and complicit in the perpetuation of the systemic violation of parents' right to informed consent by state governments.

Take Monahan's reliance on Dr. Gorski to make her case. She described him as the editor of a science journal, but the journal that she was referring to is Gorski's personal blog. Gorski is widely known among members of the health freedom movement, which he fallaciously mischaracterizes as "the anti-vaccine movement," for being an outspoken apologist for public vaccine policy whose attacks on informed-consent advocates are characterized by fallacies such as ad hominem and strawman argumentation.

An example of Gorski's typical strawman argumentation is conveniently provided for us right in the *Willamette Week* article. Contrary to Gorski's scornful personal attack, Thomas does *not* claim that children today are not healthier than they were, say, at the start of the twentieth century. Rather, what Thomas *correctly* observes is that there have been alarming increases in the rates of chronic diseases and disorders over the past several decades coinciding with the increasing number of vaccines on the CDC's schedule.

Monahan also relied on Dr. Rosenbloom as though he were merely an objective expert observer. She failed to disclose that Rosenbloom had a conflict of interest as someone with a personal stake in maintaining existing public policy. Specifically, *Rosenbloom had sponsored and submitted the 2013 legislation making it harder for parents to obtain a "nonmedical" exemption by requiring them to receive a state-approved "education" about vaccines.*[7]

The information parents get from Boost Oregon, the organization Rosenbloom is also affiliated with, is similar to the information they receive from the state's online "education" module: it is transparently intended *not* to provide parents with the knowledge they need to make an informed choice but to persuade them into compliance, including by *misinforming* parents about what science says about vaccine safety and effectiveness.

Boost Oregon *falsely* claims, for example, that aluminum and ethylmercury from vaccines are readily eliminated and do not accumulate in the body. Illustrating how misinformation from the CDC is accepted unquestioningly by most within the medical community, the group supports its claim about mercury by citing the CDC's webpage that in turn cites the 2004 Institute of Medicine review describing thimerosal as "a known neurotoxin" that "accumulates in the brain" and the 2005 study expressing concern that the neuroinflammatory process associated with mercury accumulation in the brain is a trait seen in patients with autism.[8]

Dr. Thomas is simply not among these kinds of doctors who unthinkingly accept the CDC's word as gospel truth and refuse to do their own research, *such as by simply examining the CDC's own sources to verify whether its claims accurately represent the science.*

Nowhere in the article did Monahan quote Thomas stating that vaccines cause autism or otherwise present any evidence to support the claim that this is what he tells parents. Thomas was presented as merely explaining his experiences with autistic patients that led him to question what he'd been told and that compelled him to open Integrative Pediatrics with informed consent as its founding principle.

Monahan also led *Willamette Week* readers to the conclusion that the boy who got tetanus was unvaccinated because he was Dr. Thomas's patient. But that is false. *Thomas never saw the boy until after he was discharged from the hospital.* The call from the family that Thomas said he'd received occurred *after* the boy was hospitalized. Thomas says that the *reason* the family called him was because the hospital would not allow them to take the boy home until they could show that the boy had a primary care physician, *and no other doctors would accept the boy into their practice due to their choice not to vaccinate.*

Ironically, the article contradicted its own central accusation against Thomas with the passing acknowledgment that Integrative Pediatrics had acquired more than 15,000 patients because "When Oregon parents want a doctor *who won't push vaccines,* Thomas is whom they see." (Emphasis added.)

In other words, parents go to see Dr. Paul because most other pediatricians try to pressure them into vaccinating strictly according to the CDC's schedule. They go to see Dr. Paul precisely because he *isn't* one of the bullies.

The message that the Oregon Medical Board has sent to all physicians in the state is that pushing parents into strict compliance with "standard of care" is bullying for which the state government is giving its full approval.

The message delivered is that *if doctors instead practice informed consent, they will be stripped of their medical license.*

While CDC Stalls, Independent Researchers Forge Ahead

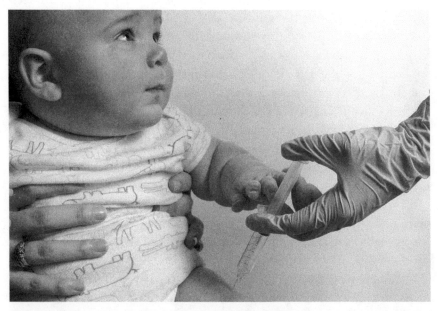

A baby receives an intramuscular vaccination in his right thigh *(public domain photo by Amanda Mills, CDC, courtesy of Pixnio).*[1]

While the CDC was still busy studying how to do a study that would suffice as the closest approximation of the type that parents were demanding, independent researchers were forging ahead with exploring observational data.

In April 2017, a pilot study was published in the *Journal of Translational Science* comparing a broad range of health outcomes between vaccinated and unvaccinated children. Since finding a study population with a sufficient proportion of unvaccinated children was otherwise a major challenge, given very high vaccination rates in the United States, the researchers looked to homeschooled children, a higher proportion of whom tend to be unvaccinated than publicly schooled children.

They gathered data by surveying mothers belonging to homeschool organizations in four states, including Oregon. Their convenience sample of 666 children included 261 who were unvaccinated. They found that unvaccinated children were less likely to have been diagnosed with allergies and neurodevelopmental disorders, with "an apparent synergistic increase" in the odds of a neurodevelopmental disorder if the child had a preterm birth.[2]

This provided concerning but inconclusive evidence that unvaccinated children might be healthier. The small sample size meant it was underpowered to detect associations with rare harms. The reliance on a survey introduced the risk of "recall bias." Parents of children who aren't vaccinated might engage in other behaviors that could potentially explain the observed association, including different health care usage leading to underdiagnosis. Given the risk of selection bias, the findings cannot be generalized to the broader population.

The study was nevertheless a step forward into the scientific void, identifying problems needing to be overcome and suggesting areas and means for further research.

Dr. Paul Thomas was also among those forging ahead, in collaboration with research scientist Dr. James Lyons-Weiler, founder of the Institute for Pure and Applied Knowledge (IPAK) and author of the book *The Environmental and Genetic Causes of Autism*.[3]

Thomas was coauthor of a study published in the *Journal of Trace Elements in Medicine and Biology* on December 5, 2019, titled "Acute exposure and chronic retention of aluminum in three vaccine schedules and effects of genetic and environmental variation." He and researchers from IPAK compared the acute exposure to aluminum that children receive from the CDC's schedule with that from Dr. Thomas's vaccine-friendly plan, which aims to reduce exposure by choosing versions that have a lower dose of aluminum, if available, and otherwise spacing vaccines out so that only one aluminum-containing vaccine is given at a time.

Noting that the government's claim that the cumulative exposure from vaccines is "safe" rests on studies of aluminum levels in the blood, they observed that this "offers little useful information to toxicology" because blood levels are not a good indicator of the amount of aluminum retained in the tissues and organs: "Thus, rapid serum or blood clearance rates can be misleadingly reassuring when considering chronic or even acute toxicity of aluminum injected with vaccines."[4]

They cited prior research showing that, contrary to popular claims, "human infants have higher exposure to aluminum from vaccination than from food, water, and formula." Their own calculations "confirm that for the CDC schedule, infants up to six months of life receive most of their metabolically available aluminum from vaccines."[5]

Furthermore, the FDA's "minimum safe level" was based on aluminum dose for adults, which was corrected by a prior study by IPAK researchers whose calculations represented "the only available dose limit for human infants that considers body weight." While no individual vaccine violated the FDA's guidance of a maximum "safe" exposure for adults, "because of multiple vaccines typically given together at 2, 4, and 6 months, the CDC schedule violates this limit even assuming an adult weight. Adjusting the safe dose limit based on a child's weight at these ages therefore results in doses that far exceed the estimated safe limit of acute toxicity."[6]

Also, the FDA's guidance did not consider chronic toxicity due to *accumulation* of aluminum from the CDC's schedule, and "[t]here are no good data available on how the retention of subsequent doses of aluminum is impacted by aluminum already in the body." The most applicable study was of aluminum retention in seven adults measuring excretion in urine, which showed that "approximately 5% of the original aluminum remains in the body of an adult a year after the dose". There were also other important considerations, "such as genetic deficiency in aluminum clearance".[7]

On all days of vaccination, the safe limit for a child was exceeded by both the CDC's schedule and the vaccine-friendly plan, which "points to acute toxicity". The CDC's schedule was the worse violator, exposing children to *nearly sixteen times the weight-adjusted recommended safe level.*

Using the best available data, they calculated that, for the CDC's schedule, "a child will be over the safe level of aluminum in the body for 149 days from birth to 7 months, constituting about 70% of days in this period. This points to chronic toxicity."

Vaccines are also only one source of aluminum exposure to consider. As they wrote, "We cannot stress how important it is that infants avoid

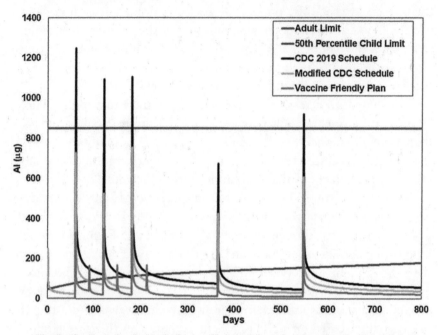

Fig. 2. Aluminum Content in Body over First Two Years for Three Vaccine Schedules.

Figure 2 from the study "Acute exposure and chronic retention of aluminum in three vaccine schedules and effects of genetic and environmental variation" compares the cumulative levels of aluminum exposure from the CDC's schedule with Dr. Paul Thomas's vaccine-friendly plan.

aluminum from all sources, at all doses, due to the realities of cumulative risk from cumulative exposure. Selecting brands of vaccines that contain lower amounts of aluminum and avoiding the combination vaccines that have the greatest amounts of aluminum would be advisable for reducing toxicity."

They strongly urged the FDA to update their guidance by establishing age-specific limits of aluminum exposure from all sources.[8]

In May 2020, a study by Brian S. Hooker and Neil Z. Miller was published in the journal *SAGE Open Medicine* comparing diagnosed health outcomes of children who were born into one of three pediatric practices and were either vaccinated or not vaccinated during their first year of life. They had a relatively high proportion of unvaccinated children in the study, which was likely a consequence of the practices respecting

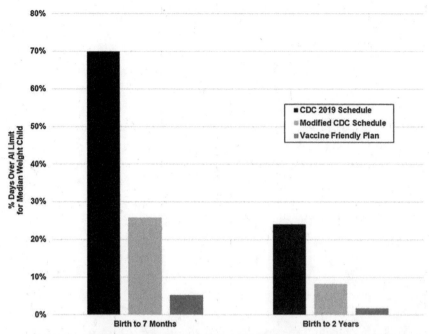

Fig. 3. Percent Days Over aluminum Limit (*%alumTox*) Birth to 7 Months and 2 Years.

Figure 3 from the study shows the percentage of days during early childhood in which the body burden of aluminum in children exceeds the corrected minimum safe level, comparing the CDC's schedule and Dr. Paul Thomas's vaccine-friendly plan.

informed consent. Specifically, they "accepted unvaccinated and partially vaccinated children into their case load".[9]

What they found was that vaccination during the first year of life was associated with twice the odds of being diagnosed for developmental delays and ear infections and over four times the odds for asthma.

When doing a quartile analysis based on the number of vaccines received (with combination vaccines being counted as a single vaccine), the pattern was one of peaking during the second or third quartiles for asthma and developmental delays, respectively. They commented that "[t]his may indicate the presence of 'healthy user bias' within the overall sample where healthy subjects continue to vaccinate but subjects with health issues limit or curtail further vaccination," as had previously been observed by researchers. "In other words, healthier vaccinated children are more likely to stay 'up-to-date' with vaccinations, whereas children showing health issues may opt for a delayed schedule or to skip specific vaccines."

This bias was minimized by directly comparing the number of vaccine doses through quartiles with outcomes for completely unvaccinated children. While the "healthy user" effect would bias their findings in favor of finding children who receive the most vaccines to have the least odds of diagnoses, there was also the potential for other confounding factors to bias their results in favor of finding unvaccinated children to be those at lowest odds of receiving a diagnosis. Nevertheless, as they commented, for some confounder to explain their increased odds of diagnosis, "it would need to be twice as frequent in vaccinated children."

They identified the main limitation of their study as being the use of a convenience sample from three practices whose pediatric populations were not characteristic of the general childhood population in the United States. Vaccine uptake was relatively low, with 30.9 percent of the sample receiving no vaccines before age one. The incidence of diagnosed autism in the study population was 0.5 percent compared with the national estimate of 1.7 percent. The incidence of diagnosed ADD or ADHD was 0.7 percent compared to the national estimate of 9 percent.[10]

One theoretical explanation for their findings is that the unvaccinated children had just as much incidence of ear infections, asthma, and developmental delays, but that they were less likely to be diagnosed because parents who decline all vaccines are less likely to take their children in to see a doctor. On the other hand, if we assume that such parents do utilize health care less frequently, it does not necessarily mean that their children are equally unhealthy but underdiagnosed. The possibility remains that their children really are generally healthier than children whose parents vaccinate to one extent or another.

Accordingly, the authors called for further research to be done using larger sample populations from a variety of pediatric practices.

Measuring the Wrong
Health Outcomes

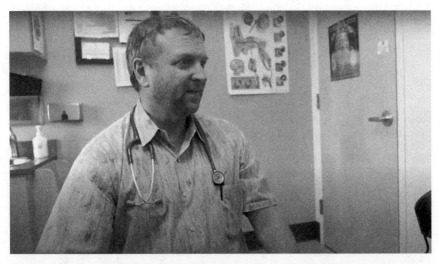

Dr. Paul Thomas with a patient in his clinic, Integrative Pediatrics *(image from "A Crazy Day in the LIfe of a Busy Pediatrician" on Dr. Paul's YouTube channel)*[1]

The complaints that the Oregon Medical Board sent to Dr. Paul Thomas were not the only actions taken against him by the state. In July 2019, shortly prior to the publication of the study showing that the vaccine-friendly plan exposed children to considerably less aluminum than the CDC's schedule, the Oregon Health Authority removed Integrative Pediatrics from the Vaccines For Children (VFC) program, which directs tax dollars toward funding childhood vaccinations for low-income families, such as those eligible for Medicaid. Under the VFC, the CDC purchases vaccines at a discount from the pharmaceutical companies and distributes them to state health departments and local public health agencies.[2]

Willamette Week ran an article about this under the headline "Vaccine-Doubting Oregon Doctor Loses Medicaid Funding." The state's ostensible reason for this action, according to the report, was that "Thomas failed to stock two of the required vaccines (the rotavirus and HPV vaccines), as mandated under the program." Asked to comment for the article, Thomas said, "I didn't jump through their hoops fast enough."[3]

During our interview, Thomas acknowledged that he did not stock those vaccines for a time for the simple reason that there was no market demand for them. Parents who chose those vaccines for their children tended instead to go to one of the many other locations where they were readily available. He said that he has stocked the vaccines in recent years for the rare occasions that parents wanted them. In a letter to the medical board, he noted that the vaccines were in inventory at the time the state terminated his practice from the VCP.[4]

Having known since the day he published *The Vaccine-Friendly Plan* that the state would go after him for not adhering to dogma, Thomas had obtained institutional review board approval to use the deidentified data from his practice for research and publication. Working again with James Lyons-Weiler, he was conducting the study to compare health outcomes between his vaccinated and unvaccinated patients.

Shortly before the study's publication, a major private provider also dropped his clinic from their coverage. Thomas says he was working on resolving the dispute with the company until the medical board issued its "emergency" suspension order.

The company cited his "alternative vaccination schedule" and the state's termination of his practice from the VCP as the main reasons for its decision, asserting that "[t]here is overwhelming evidence that childhood vaccines are safe and effective."[5]

Thomas thinks that he was dropped because one of their "quality measures" is vaccination rates, the assumption being that a lower vaccination rate indicates inferior care. He gave the example of the Hepatitis B (HepB) vaccine, which is routinely administered to babies on the very first day of their lives.

Thomas described the CDC recommendation for *universal* HepB vaccination at birth as "insanity." As he correctly pointed out, this virus is typically transmitted through sexual intercourse or shared needles among intravenous drug users. The risk to infants comes from the small percentage of mothers who are carriers, but routine screening is done during pregnancy to determine whether this is a risk. Consequently, for infants whose mothers are not carriers, the adjuvanted HepB vaccine is an unnecessary exposure to aluminum.

Indeed, the CDC's stated rationale for administering this vaccine at birth is simply that there was insufficient demand for it among sexually active adults and intravenous drug addicts, and so the determination was made to vaccinate all babies at birth to achieve the policy goal of greater vaccine uptake.

In the CDC's own words, the problem that this 1991 recommendation was intended to overcome was that "[i]n the United States, most infections occur among adults and adolescents. The recommended strategy for preventing these infections has been the selective vaccination of persons with identified risk factors. However, the strategy has not lowered the incidence of hepatitis B, primarily because vaccinating persons engaged in high-risk behaviors, lifestyles, or occupations before they become infected generally has not been feasible."[6]

Since many parents in his practice decline this vaccine, his vaccination rate is lower, and therefore he is not meeting their standards. But he takes issue with their standards, arguing that they measure the wrong outcome.

"We shouldn't be looking at how well somebody can follow a protocol," Thomas said. "Monkeys can do that. We should be looking at actual health outcomes, which is what our study did. So, I think that that's part of the problem here."

He added, "My duty is to my patients, and we have a lot of loyal patients who, you know, love the fact that we honor and provide informed consent and provide great care, and we have great outcomes, which are now documented in a published peer-reviewed study."

The study was published on November 22, 2020. In it, Dr. Thomas and Dr. Lyons-Weiler compared incidence of diagnoses of a wide range of health problems and found that the completely unvaccinated children in his practice were diagnosed at much lower rates. While incidence of diagnosis is a commonly used measure in observational vaccine safety studies, it indicates only whether a patient has the condition. It says nothing about its *severity*. So, they also developed a new methodology to measure incidence of office visits for each negative health outcome.

"This study represents a major methodological leap forward in vaccine safety studies," said Lyons-Weiler on the IPAK website. "The results show how often vaccinating patients have to seek medical care for conditions suspected by many as potentially caused by vaccines. Our measure, the Relative Incidence of Office Visits (RIOV), is sensitive to the severity of disease and disorder—specifically, the disease burden."

They note that the study does *not* prove that vaccines *caused* the negative health outcomes. However, they did attempt to account for differences in health care usage that might confound their findings.

"While teasing out causality is difficult in observational studies," said Lyons-Weiler, "our use of natural internal positive and negative control conditions—fever, which is known to be caused by vaccines, and well-baby visits, which is not caused by vaccines—provide added assurance that we are seeing a likely causal signature."[7]

Just eleven days after the study was published, on December 3, 2020, the CDC published an update on its progress in determining how to use the Vaccine Safety Datalink to help answer the primary question, "How do child health outcomes compare between those who receive no vaccinations and those who receive the full currently recommended immunization schedule?"

Comparing rates of health care utilization between "undervaccinated" and "age-appropriately vaccinated" children, they found that children who were "undervaccinated" due to parental choice "had lower rates of outpatient visits and emergency department encounters".

Included under the label "undervaccinated" were the approximately 1 percent of children for whom there was no record of receiving any recommended vaccinations during the first two years of life.

The CDC document cited several prior VSD studies assessing various negative health outcomes. None of them compared health outcomes between children vaccinated according to the CDC's schedule and unvaccinated children.[8]

The very same day, the Oregon Medical Board issued its order to suspend Dr. Thomas's license on the grounds of a public health "emergency."

It was indeed an emergency for public health authorities, whose credibility was sorely damaged by the published data showing that Dr. Thomas achieves superior health outcomes with the pediatric patients in his practice.

How the Media Reported Dr. Paul's Suspension

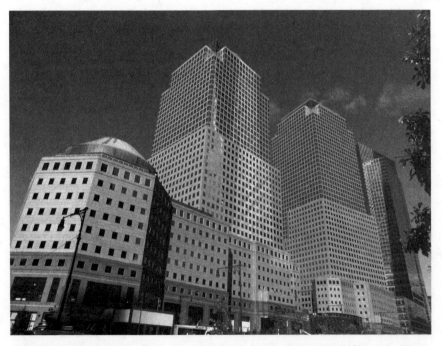

200 Liberty Street, New York, New York, where the Associated Press is head-quartered *(photo by giggel, licensed under CC BY 3.0)*[1]

Media reports have unquestioningly characterized the Oregon Medical Board's suspension of Dr. Thomas's license as justified. *Willamette Week* on December 6 described him as "a prominent anti-vaccine pediatrician", notwithstanding the fact that he vaccinated patients in his practice or that his own children were vaccinated. Dr. Thomas, the article uncritically parroted, "had violated standard medical practices related to vaccines."

The newspaper also observed that the first complaint listed by the medical board matched the details of Leah Klass's accusation against Thomas in the same newspaper in March 2019, which was written by the same reporter, Rachel Monahan.

A second allegation contained in the board's suspension order also echoed the newspaper's prior reporting. "Thomas also was a doctor of a high-profile patient," Monahan wrote, "who contracted tetanus on a farm and spent two months in an intensive care unit, *WW* reported in 2019. But the medical board order includes a new detail: that he apparently saw the patient for follow-up care."[2]

This again misled the public to the *false* conclusion that the boy had not been vaccinated because he was a patient of Dr. Thomas's, when in fact Thomas never saw the boy until *after* his discharge from the hospital, which resulted specifically because the boy's parents were already determined not to vaccinate him and could find no other pediatricians who would take the boy into their practice.

According to Thomas, with reference to the boy's treatment for tetanus at the Oregon Health & Science University Hospital, "The family contacted Integrative Pediatrics in despair since OHSU would not discharge them until they found a pediatrician *and* they could not find any office willing to take them given their prior refusal of vaccines."

The similarly misleading headline of an OregonLive article read, "Anti-vaccine Portland pediatrician's license suspended; cases include boy hospitalized with tetanus". The lead paragraph furthered the deception by stating that the board had cited "a litany of cases in which he failed to adequately vaccinate patients, including a case involving a boy who contracted tetanus and required hospitalization for 57 days."[3]

On Twitter, the author of the OregonLive article, Lizzy Acker, shared the piece with the remark: "Remember the kid who was hospitalized for two months with tetanus and then his parents still didn't vaccinate him? His doctor's license was suspended last week."[4]

Neither *Willamette Week* nor OregonLive reported that Dr. Thomas had just published a study in a peer-reviewed journal showing that, if anything, his unvaccinated children were *healthier* than those who had been vaccinated to one extent or another.

I confronted Acker about this on Twitter, asking her if she was aware of the study and noting that this fact was highly relevant and should be reported. I provided the link to the study.[5] Thomas's coauthor on the study, Dr. James Lyons-Weiler, responded to Acker in turn by stating, "This was retaliation for a study they wanted. The medical board has declared war on objective Science and on Informed Consent. There is much more to this story. Please investigate."[6]

We received no reply to our mutual request for her to do real journalism as opposed to propagandizing for the state.

Incidentally, the deceptive OregonLive piece represented a reversal of opinion about Dr. Thomas. Back in 2009, the paper had done a flattering story on him titled "Love builds the Thomas family: from Africa to Portland, from five kids to nine."[7]

The story about the medical board's suspension of Thomas was carried nationally by the Associated Press (AP), which similarly propagated the deception by saying in its lead paragraph that the board had cited "multiple cases in which he allegedly failed to adequately vaccinate patients, including one involving a child who contracted tetanus and required hospitalization."

The AP said that the board had "found" that Thomas "had a history of misleading parents" about vaccines, as though this were a proven fact rather than an accusation by the state for which there was an obvious political motive and no credible supporting evidence. There was also no mention in the AP report of the study showing that Dr. Thomas's unvaccinated patients were considerably less likely to be diagnosed with a broad range of health problems.[8]

Thomas doesn't think that the timing of the board's "emergency" suspension order was a coincidence. He was due to give the board some information that it had requested about the sales of his book *The Vaccine-Friendly Plan* later that same week. "What does that have to do with anything?" he asked rhetorically, suggesting that they were "fishing" for anything they could use to come after him. But why wouldn't they have waited for that information? What had changed? Why had the board's interest in him gone from an ongoing inquiry suddenly to an "emergent" need to suspend his license?

The only thing that changed, he said, was that their study was published: "This paper is very threatening to the status quo, to the entire vaccine industry that wants to continue spouting off their mantra, their marketing slogan that 'vaccines are safe and effective.' That's clear as the light of day."

The timing certainly does suggest retaliation for threatening the status quo and the credibility of public health authorities not only in Oregon, but in other states as well as the federal government. And the board's suspension order did not specify anything else that had changed that would warrant suspending his license *before* their investigation into his practice was concluded.

Indeed, the board's perceived need to suspend his license "while this case remains under investigation" strongly suggests that the outcome of that investigation was being prejudged *precisely* because the data that the board had *asked* Thomas to produce might lead not only to his being absolved of wrongdoing but also to the authorities losing credibility in the eyes of the public. Clearly, there was an emergent need to act preemptively to punish him and, in so doing, to prejudice public opinion against him.[9]

The Oregon Medical Board's Accusations

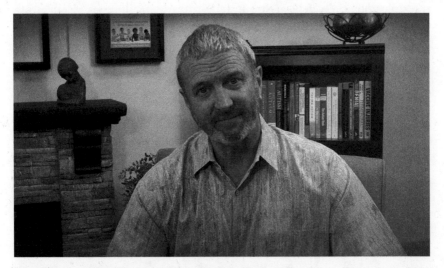

Paul Thomas, MD, discusses the Oregon Medical Board's suspension of his license in a video on his YouTube channel.[1]

The "emergency" suspension order issued by the Oregon Medical Board on December 3, 2020, alleged that Dr. Thomas's "continued practice constitutes an immediate danger to the public" and "a serious danger to the public health or safety." The CDC's routine childhood vaccine schedule, the board stated, "has been relied upon for many years" and "is widely accepted as authoritative in the medical community." It was the "standard of care in Oregon."

The core accusation was that, by having lower than expected vaccination rates among his patients, Thomas had "breached the standard of
care" and thereby "placed the health and safety of many of his patients
at serious risk of harm." This was the reason provided by the board for
declaring that it was "therefore necessary to emergently suspend Licensee's
license to practice medicine."

The board claimed that Thomas "promotes his unique, 'Dr. Paul
approved' schedule as providing superior results to any other option,
namely improved health on many measures, and fraudulently asserts that
following his vaccine schedule will prevent or decrease the incidence of
autism and other developmental disorders."

Thomas used that claim, according to the board, "to solicit parental
'refusal' of full vaccination for their children, thereby exposing them to
multiple potentially debilitating and life-threatening illnesses". Reiterating
its accusation, the board accused that his "promotion of this alternative
vaccination schedule exposes patients to the risk of harm in violation of
ORS 677.190(1)(a), as defined by ORS 677.188(4)(a)." Thomas "is insistent
and direct in his communication with parents and guardians", the board
accused, "that they should accept his alternative vaccine schedule."[2]

The statutes cited state that the Oregon Medical Board may suspend or revoke a license to practice for "[u]nprofessional or dishonorable
conduct." This is defined as "conduct unbecoming a person licensed to
practice medicine . . . or detrimental to the best interests of the public,"
including any "conduct or practice contrary to recognized standards of
ethics of the medical . . . profession or any conduct or practice which
does or might constitute a danger to the health or safety of a patient or
the public".[3]

Thomas maintains that these accusations demonstrate that the medical board fails to even comprehend the concept of informed consent and
consequently has no idea how things are done in his practice. He does
not tell his patients what to do one way or the other. He discusses the
CDC's recommendations and provides other information so that parents
can make their own educated decision.

The law explicitly allows for use of "alternative medical treatment",
the definition of which includes treatment "that the treating physician,
based on the physician's professional experience, has an objective basis to
believe has a reasonable probability for effectiveness in its intended use

even if the treatment is outside recognized scientific guidelines" or "is unproven".[4]

Thomas denies that he tells parents that the vaccine-friendly plan is superior to other schedules. On the contrary, to suggest that all patients strictly comply with this alternative schedule *would be contrary to the whole concept*, which is that a risk-benefit analysis must be done for each vaccine and each child so that the approach with respect to vaccination is tailored to the health needs of the individual. He *rejects* the CDC's one-size-fits-all approach and, contrary to the board's allegation, does *not* take that same approach with the vaccine-friendly plan.

"The truth is I am the only full-service medical home pediatric clinic that honors informed consent," Thomas said, "and that seems to be a threat to the establishment that wants one-size-fits-all medicine."

He added, "I still can't quite figure out what the 'emergency' is. Maybe I'll be giving more informed consent. I guess that's a threat. Seriously, that's the only thing they can charge me with that stands and that's true, is that I give informed consent."

Furthermore, Thomas denies that he tells parents that vaccines cause autism. Rather, he considers it unethical to explain only the benefits of vaccines without also discussing potential risks. He therefore relates the observations of other parents as well as his own experience of witnessing children regress into autism after vaccination, as well as his observation that patients whose parents opted for a personalized schedule and carefully limited aluminum exposure each visit have generally had better health outcomes.

That observation of his, he notes, is now well supported by a peer-reviewed study.

To support its accusation that Dr. Thomas had behaved unprofessionally, the board cited several patient cases, each of which warrants examination.

Patient A: Mom Accuses Dr. Paul of "Bullying"

The first case presented as evidence against Thomas was that of "Patient A," whose mother had left his practice for another provider "after having been 'reduced to tears' by Licensee's 'bullying' her into his personal vaccine schedule against her express wishes for full vaccination for her child."

According to the mother, she "requested polio and rotavirus vaccinations", but Thomas "did not have those vaccines in the clinic". She also claimed that he "questioned why she wanted Patient A to get the polio vaccine and asked whether they were traveling to Africa. During the appointment, Licensee continually connected vaccines (not specific) with autism. Licensee asked her how awful she would feel if Patient A got autism and she could have prevented it."

As far as the Oregon Medical Board was concerned, the mother's accusation was sufficient to conclude that Thomas had made "false claims regarding the safety of the CDC Recommendations". The board declared that his "failure" to vaccinate the child according to CDC's schedule "absent unsolicited parental refusal, his failure to document any such refusal, and his failure to adequately vaccinate children is grossly negligent".

This is the mother whose allegation the *Willamette Week* said matches the public allegation made by Leah Klass. While it is possible that the board was referring to a different woman, the similarity to Klass's accusation does suggest that she was the source of this claim.

It is obvious that the Oregon Medical Board has no problem with pediatricians bullying or otherwise pressuring parents into vaccinating their children strictly according to the CDC's schedule, including by threatening to kick them out of the practice for declining.

Setting aside the rank hypocrisy, we can stipulate that it would be unprofessional for Dr. Thomas to bully parents into choosing his vaccine-friendly plan. But did he?

As noted, when the *Willamette Week* first reported Leah Klass's accusation, Thomas denied that it had ever happened. He also described the characterization of the conversation presented by the medical board as "false".

When asked if he had ever had a parent say that they want to vaccinate according to the CDC's schedule but he tried to persuade them not to, Thomas replied:

> No, I think that's too strong of a statement, "to persuade." My role is to inform, and they're the ones who have do decide. Now, I think it gets a little gray in the case of, uh—here's where it gets difficult: we have situations, and it happens more often than I'd like to say—I mean maybe two or three times a year—that are extraordinarily difficult because you have one

parent who wants to follow the CDC schedule, and you have one parent who doesn't want to do any.

That situation happens once in a while, and it is an absolute no-win situation because they're at odds, so I don't want to take sides. It's a parental decision. So, what happens in those situations is that as I go through the information so they can make an informed decision, the parent who wants to do all the vaccines doesn't feel supported because I'm *also* giving information that relates to harm from vaccines, and that challenges their beliefs, and they get mad.

He initially thought the incident described with "Patient A" might have been such a case. He recalled a time when a mother did storm out in tears:

One of my nurse practitioners was seeing that couple, and she came to me saying, "I don't know what to do. The mom wants to do all of them, and I don't know if the dad is on the same page." And she was distraught, right? And she just really didn't know what to do. And I said, "Oh, I'll take care of it," and I walked in blind. And I'm used to dealing with these things, and I didn't realize the tension level in that room was already thick, so, "Hey, I'm trying to help you out, figure out what to do about vaccines."

"Well, I just want to do them all. I don't know what the problem is." Something like that.

"Okay, okay, I just want to have a discussion." And I turned to the dad, and I said, "Are you guys on the same page?"

Well, basically, that just infuriated this mom. She jumped out of her seat and just stormed out in tears. I mean, it happened really fast.

After reviewing the details of the described incident and his patient records, he concluded that was not the same mom whose complaint was included in the medical board's suspension order. To the best that he has been able to determine, the source of the allegation is a mom whose baby he had seen only twice, for the newborn and two-month well visits, in 2013.

Having consulted his records, he said that the mother consented to DTaP and *Haemophilus influenzae type b* (Hib) vaccinations but *did* sign a declination form for hepatitis B, polio, rotavirus, and pneumococcal vaccines. He does not practice "medical shaming"; he practices informed consent. He said he cannot recall a time in the past thirteen years when he did not have the polio vaccine available, although he acknowledges there was a period when he did not stock the rotavirus vaccine due to lack of demand.

Notably, the rotavirus vaccine is not required by the state of Oregon for children to attend school.[5]

With respect to the polio vaccine, Thomas also noted that it is pertinent to ask whether the patient is traveling to a location where the poliovirus is still present since it has been eradicated from the United States and most other countries.

He said he does not recall that mother being tearful, and he wonders why a parent who didn't care to be fully informed would choose to go to his clinic since he was well known in the community for uniquely providing individualized care in accordance with his legal obligation to obtain informed consent.

Patient B: Older Brother with Pertussis

The remainder of the medical board's allegations revolved around what the suspension order describes as "unprofessional or dishonorable conduct which exposed his patients to the risk of harm, as well as gross or repeated acts of negligence".

On its face, this overlooks the fact that the choice to vaccinate is *also* a choice to expose the child to the risk of harm. It is as though the Oregon Medical Board does not even understand the concept of an individual risk-benefit analysis and is assuming that vaccinations are all benefit and no risk for everybody.

The next two cases that the board presented to support the allegation were brothers, one aged eleven years and the other aged seven years. According to the medical board, the elder, "Patient B," was vaccinated "on a delayed schedule according to Licensee's recommendations and practice agreements" and "was subsequently diagnosed with pertussis on September 24, 2018, requiring office visits and antibiotics."

In this context, the board claimed that "Pertussis is a fully vaccine-preventable illness." It also claimed that the boy's chart showed that he was not vaccinated for pertussis, "but there are no records of recommendation for immunization or parental refusal of vaccines."[6]

The board's allegation makes it sound as though parents who would like for Dr. Thomas to be their child's pediatrician must sign a "practice agreement" to accept a "delayed schedule", but this is untrue. Thomas said that the only thing that fits the description of a "practice agreement" is the formal process by which informed consent is obtained or declination is documented.

He also said that the claim that there is no such record for the boy is false. The well-child visits were conducted by other practitioners in his clinic, and a review of his records showed that the parents affirmed declination on April 2, 2014; August 19, 2015; and April 15, 2020. He said the Oregon Medical Board is in possession of these records and that the family was still with the practice.

The board's claim that pertussis is a "fully vaccine-preventable illness" is also demonstrably false—a statement of *faith*, not science.

As the *New York Times* reported in 2015, since 2008, the greatest risk to infants of being infected with the bacterium that causes "whooping cough" comes from their older siblings, not from the parents, as had historically been the case.

In the past, most children would have been naturally exposed to pertussis and developed a robust immunity lasting until their adulthood. The shift, the *Times* acknowledged, was "probably a result of waning immunity among children and adolescents who had received the DTaP vaccine."

As the *Times* admitted, "the disease can spread from vaccinated siblings" to infants too young to be vaccinated, who are at higher risk from the disease.[7]

In fact, studies show that vaccine-conferred immunity to pertussis may wane in as few as two to three years, which helps explain the resurgence of whooping cough in countries where the acellular pertussis vaccine is recommended for routine use in children. Additionally, the vaccine does not confer mucosal immunity or other cellular immune responses in the same way that occurs with natural immunity, and, consequently, the vaccine does not prevent transmission of pertussis.[8]

As the FDA acknowledged in 2013, while individuals who receive the pertussis vaccine "may be protected from disease, they may still become infected with the bacteria without always getting sick and are able to spread infection to others, including young infants."[9]

The *New York Times* at the time quoted the lead author of that FDA study saying, "When you're newly vaccinated you are an asymptomatic carrier, which is good for you, but not for the population."[10]

In contrast to the Oregon Medical Board's claim that pertussis is "fully vaccine-preventable", a study published in the journal *Clinical*

Infectious Diseases in 2015 observed that it was "the least well-controlled vaccine-preventable disease despite excellent vaccination coverage and 6 vaccine doses recommended between 2 months of age and adolescence."[11]

That is to say, "undervaccination" is emphatically *not* the problem.

Additionally, waning immunity and failure to prevent transmission are not the only factors contributing to the problem. Mass vaccination itself appears to have put evolutionary pressure on pertussis bacteria so that, today, the variants in circulation have adapted to escape vaccine-conferred immunity.

As a review published in *Tropical Diseases, Travel Medicine and Vaccines* in 2016 observed, "Just as exposure to antibiotics creates a selective evolutionary pressure for bacteria to develop resistance to antibiotics, so too can vaccines exert pressure for bacteria to evolve to different antigenic isoforms of proteins included in vaccines."[12]

Such adaptation "has been clearly demonstrated to occur" with the pertussis vaccine. While there are a number of explanatory mechanisms, the most "definitive evolutionary escape route" has been the selection of strains lacking expression of antigen genes entirely. Most remarkably, the review authors stated, strains expressing the protein pertactin (PRN), which is a key antigen component of the vaccine, "have entirely disappeared from the US".[13]

The CDC had acknowledged in 2012 that data from Washington and Vermont showed that "85% of the isolates were PRN-deficient" and, moreover, that "vaccinated patients had significantly higher odds than unvaccinated patients of being infected with PRN-deficient strains", which suggested that pertactin-deficient bacteria "may have a selective advantage in infecting DTaP-vaccinated persons."[14]

As already noted, a study published in 2019 concluded that "all children who were primed by DTaP vaccines will be more susceptible to pertussis throughout their lifetimes".[15]

In short, the Oregon Medical Board's claim that pertussis is "fully vaccine-preventable" is irreconcilable with the science and simply illustrates the extraordinary ignorance and hypocrisy of its members.

Patient C: Younger Brother with Pertussis

The third patient was the younger brother of Patient B. In August 2013, at ten weeks of age, the younger sibling was admitted to the hospital with a fever and diagnosed with Kawasaki disease. Dr. Thomas had seen the boy for three days in the clinic with a fever and treated him with an antibiotic "on the basis of a 'bagged' and not catharized urine sample and in the absence of blood cultures." The board's accusation is that Thomas "breached the standard of care" by failing to refer the patient to the hospital for diagnostic testing.

A second accusation in this case is that the boy did not receive the pertussis vaccine "and subsequently contracted pertussis" when his older brother had it in September 2018.[16]

The board's suggestion that a fever lasting three days was not only cause for Dr. Thomas to refer the boy to the hospital but also grounds for suspending his license for not having done so is inconsistent with the advice that Mayo Clinic gives to parents whose child has a fever. The recommendation is that parents should take their child in to see their child's doctor if the fever lasts "longer than three days".[17]

This raises the question of why, if a fever lasting no more than three days is insufficient cause for parents to take their child in to their pediatrician, a pediatrician should be stripped of his license for not referring the parents to the hospital within that same period.

Mayo Clinic's page on Kawasaki disease states that its symptoms may include a high fever that "lasts for more than three days", which likewise raises the question of why a pediatrician should be punished for not immediately suspecting Kawasaki disease *within* that three-day period.[18]

Mayo Clinic's information on what to do about a fever also tells parents that their child's doctor "may prescribe an antibiotic, especially if he or she suspects a bacterial infection".[19]

Dr. Thomas argues that the standards of care to rule out potential causes apply to an emergency department or hospital setting for infants less than six to eight weeks of age who have a fever of unknown cause, not to an older infant in an office setting. He said that his records note that he attempted unsuccessfully to obtain a urine sample using a catheter, so he then tried successfully using the other method. He insists that the care the child received was appropriate for the situation.

Suspecting a urinary tract infection, he treated with an antibiotic while awaiting lab results from the urine specimen, and he had the patient follow up the next day. The lab results confirmed his suspicion.

Furthermore, when Thomas came to suspect Kawasaki disease, he *did* refer the patient to the hospital, where that suspicion was confirmed, too. This enabled the child to be diagnosed on a timely basis and treated with intravenous immunoglobulin to prevent potentially serious heart conditions that can occur in Kawasaki patients. He describes the child's outcome as successful.

As for the fact that the boy was unvaccinated, Dr. Thomas said that the parents signed declination forms on January 2, 2014; August 20, 2015; January 26, 2018; April 22, 2019; and most recently on May 29, 2020, during the boy's seven-year well visit.

It is also noteworthy that the pertussis vaccine is one of the shots recommended in his vaccine-friendly plan, so the board cannot possibly argue that his unvaccinated status was a result of Thomas pushing the parents to follow that schedule.

In essence, once again, the Oregon Medical Board is accusing Thomas of having respected the parents' right to informed consent rather than pressuring them to vaccinate strictly according to the CDC's schedule.

Patient D: Boy with Tetanus

The fourth case presented by the medical board is the boy who had gotten tetanus in 2017, who media reports had falsely suggested was unvaccinated by virtue of being Dr. Thomas's patient. Indeed, this false characterization of the event is precisely the picture that the Oregon Medical Board deceptively conveys.

The boy's case was described by the CDC in a report published in its *Morbidity and Mortality Weekly Report* (*MMWR*) in March 2019. At six years of age, the completely unvaccinated boy "sustained a forehead laceration while playing outdoors on a farm; the wound was cleaned and sutured at home."

At the hospital, tetanus immune globulin and a dose of pertussis vaccine were administered. The CDC notes that "Despite extensive review of the risks and benefits of tetanus vaccination by physicians, the family declined the second dose of DTaP and any other recommended immunizations."[20]

The Oregon Medical Board's suspension order relates how the boy got cut on the family farm, how the parents sutured the wound themselves, and how he was hospitalized for tetanus. Then, the board states that Dr. Thomas "saw Patient D for follow-up in clinic on November 17, 2017." It also states that Thomas "did not document an informed consent discussion about the risk/benefit of immunization". This, the board accused, "placed Patient D at serious risk of harm and constitutes gross negligence."[21]

Of course, what the Oregon Medical Board left out of its suspension order was the fact that the boy had not seen Dr. Thomas until *after* he was discharged from the hospital. The board also failed to note that the tetanus vaccine is among those recommended under the vaccine-friendly plan. Also withheld by the board was the fact that the *reason* the parents called Dr. Thomas was that other doctors wouldn't accept the boy as their patient given the parents' refusal to vaccinate him.

Notably, if we accept that failing to convince the parents to accept the second dose of the pertussis vaccine constitutes a violation of Oregon law, then we must also concede that all the doctors at the hospital who failed to get them to do so should be stripped of their licenses, too.

When Dr. Thomas saw the boy after his discharge, the parents made it clear to him that they were not going to do any more vaccinations. He says that, while he may not have pursued the paperwork on vaccine declination during that first appointment, he did so at the next well-child visit, on November 9, 2020, at which time both parents signed the declination form for all CDC-recommended vaccines.

Once again, what it comes down to is that the Oregon Medical Board has accused Dr. Paul Thomas of the grave sin of respecting his patients' right to informed consent.

Patient E: Girl with Rotavirus

The next case presented by the medical board was that of a ten-year-old girl who "received minimal immunization" in Dr. Thomas's clinic and, in April 2011, "required hospitalization for rotavirus gastroenteritis". She had also had a cough and was "treated empirically for pertussis without testing by another physician" in the clinic. The care provided to the girl, the board charged, "breached the standard of care and exposed the patient to the serious risk of harm."[22]

The CDC's schedule recommends two doses of the rotavirus vaccine at the age of two months and four months, respectively. This girl, Thomas says, was eleven months old when he first saw her as his patient. The parents signed vaccine declination forms at that first visit on January 5, 2012, and again on January 13, 2015, and March 2, 2016. While it isn't a standard procedure in his own practice, he says that physicians commonly treat cough with antibiotics. He also says that he has only had three cases of rotavirus gastroenteritis in his thirteen years at Integrative Pediatrics despite the parents of most children who were born into that practice declining the vaccine.

Additionally, the study Thomas and Lyons-Weiler published just prior to the board's suspension order shows that his unvaccinated patients have had significantly less incidence of gastroenteritis.[23]

Once again, what the Oregon Medical Board's charge appears to boil down to is that Dr. Thomas respected the parents' right to informed consent rather than doing everything in his power to coerce the parents into vaccination. It appears that the medical board is accusing Dr. Thomas of being unfit for duty because he refuses to violate Oregon law requiring him to obtain informed consent.

Patient F: Girl with Gut Problems and Allergies

The medical board described the sixth case as follows:

> Patient F is a 7-year-old female who Licensee followed in clinic for consti-
> pation, food allergies, mold allergies and possible "chronic Lyme disease.["]
> Review of her chart from Licensee's clinic reveals that she was nonimmu-
> nized. Licensee ordered repeated IgE allergy panels and recommended
> elimination diets, vitamin supplements and provided antibiotics for acute
> infections. Licensee failed to provide an appropriate referral to a pediatric
> gastroenterologist to exclude a diagnosis of malabsorption or celiac dis-
> ease, a referral to pediatric allergy/immunology or to pediatric nutrition.
> Licensee's neglect to seek consultative support and oversight, and his fail-
> ure to address Patient F's lack of immunizations, placed the health of this
> patient at serious risk and was grossly negligent.[24]

The board does not say that the girl was ever diagnosed with a disease it considers "vaccine-preventable". Dr. Thomas says this girl's parents signed declination forms on November 5, 2013; January 29, 2014; July 7, 2014; November 12, 2014; January 4, 2017; December 21, 2017; January 3, 2019; and August 19, 2020. Once again, with respect to vaccination, the medical board's charge is essentially that Dr. Thomas practiced informed consent.

Apart from that, the board seems to be accusing Dr. Thomas of considering things that most other doctors would not for the simple reason that they do not keep up with the science.

He says that the girl was also seeing a naturopath who had recommended testing for IgE-mediated allergies, and so it was by request that this was done in his clinic. Dr. Thomas says he regularly refers patients to other physicians and does not try to hamper the referrals or second opinions of others, such as by refusing to do the requested testing.

Thomas also says that he sees a lot of chronic allergy patients because specialists often refuse to acknowledge the existence of non-IgE food sensitivities and do nothing to try to identify them. He says that hundreds of patients in his clinic have successfully reduced or eliminated symptoms by identifying and eliminating trigger foods.[25]

An "elimination diet" is a useful method for identifying triggering foods that can otherwise be difficult to identify due to the oftentimes delayed reactions. The idea is to eliminate the most common culprits from the diet and then slowly reintroduce them one by one to identify those that trigger symptoms.

The existence of non-IgE-mediated allergic responses may be widely dismissed by general practitioners but is not controversial in the medical literature. A study published in *Annals of Allergy* in 1984, for example, noted that "[p]reliminary findings suggest that IgG4 antibodies may be important in certain types of food allergic reactions."[26]

A study published in *Nutrition in Clinical Practice* in 2010 observed that "[a]mong modalities used by many conventional and alternative practitioners, immunoglobulin G (IgG)-based testing showed promise, with clinically meaningful results. It has been proven useful as a guide for elimination diets, with clinical impact for a variety of diseases."[27]

A review published in the *Journal of Allergy and Clinical Immunology* in 2015 noted that among the most common non-IgE-mediated allergens are proteins in cow's milk, soy, and wheat. While noting that IgG testing is not recommended by the National Institute for Allergic and Infectious Diseases (NIAID) or allergy-focused trade organizations, an elimination diet can result in effective treatment by learning which foods to avoid, which in turn enables the chronic inflammation to subside and the mucosal lining of the gut to heal.[28]

An associated problem is that of "leaky gut," or intestinal hyperpermeability, which is known to be associated with the development of autoimmune diseases if left unresolved. A study published in *Autoimmunity Reviews* in November 2018 expressed curiosity that the medical establishment has given "so little attention" to the role of diet in the development of autoimmunity, including the role of leaky gut and exposures to pesticides, preservatives, and nutrient deficiencies.

The review found that IgG levels for specific food antibodies were "significantly higher" in patients with autoimmune disease compared to a control group without autoimmunity, while reactions to some foods was not associated with an increased level of IgG. The author concluded that, despite remaining uncertainties, IgG testing could be an important tool to help in the process of determining which foods should be avoided by patients with or at risk for autoimmune disease.[29]

A study published in *Allergy, Asthma & Clinical Immunology* in 2018, titled "non-IgE-mediated food hypersensitivity," also noted that an elimination diet was an effective approach for treating symptoms through avoidance of food triggers.[30]

A literature review published in *Current Pain and Headache Reports* in 2019 noted that "IgG food sensitivities have been linked to various symptoms and disorders" and that some evidence "supports the use of IgG food sensitivity testing". The conclusion of the review was that "IgG food sensitivity testing may prove to be a beneficial tool for healthcare practitioners, especially for patients experiencing migraine headache symptoms."[31]

A review published in July 2020 in the journal *Nutrients* observed that there is "poor familiarity" with non-IgE-mediated food allergies among health care providers, and that this "lack of awareness" is a contributing factor in the failure to diagnose and effectively treat symptoms by eliminating offending foods.[32]

In essence, the medical board is not only seeking to punish Dr. Thomas for practicing informed consent in respectful cooperation with other physicians seen by his patients, but also for keeping up to date on advances in medical science and *effectively* treating patients in ways that the medical establishment hasn't caught up with yet.

Patients G & H: Twins with Rotavirus

The final two cases that the board presented to support its accusations were twins born prematurely. They did not receive the rotavirus vaccine and at ten months of age were hospitalized for rotavirus. The board declares that they "had no chronic medical conditions that would justify medical immunization exemptions" and that the patient chart "contains documentation of parental refusal of vaccines, but they are inconsistent regarding specific vaccines and their timing." The board further claimed that "[r]otavirus infection is fully vaccine-preventable."

Additionally, the board asserted that the girls' mother "stated during hospitalization that she thought her children had received rotavirus vaccine", and it charged that "[f]ailure to document specific parental refusal and lack of providing parental clarity constitutes acts of negligence."[33]

However, as Dr. Thomas points out, the medical board's claim that rotavirus infection is "fully vaccine-preventable" is false. Children who get vaccinated can still get rotavirus, and vaccinated children can potentially spread the vaccine-strain virus to unvaccinated children.

Indeed, the rotavirus vaccine is estimated to be not 100 percent but 70 percent to 84 percent effective in preventing rotavirus-associated emergency room visits plus hospitalization.[34] A study published in *BMC Infectious Diseases* in November 2019 confirmed that vaccinated children can have symptomatic rotavirus infection, with 30 percent of children in the study who'd been diagnosed with rotavirus having been vaccinated.[35]

A study published in *Pediatrics* in 2016 noted that the prevalence of rotavirus increased with age in vaccinated children, which was "the opposite" of what was observed "in children who were unlikely to have been vaccinated" and indicated "potential waning immunity" with the vaccine. (The study also noted that, before the vaccine, rotavirus was biennial and seasonal in occurrence, and that, contrary to a "flawed" CDC report, "the length of each season in the postvaccine period increased rather than decreased as reported by the CDC for all peak seasons."[36])

While in developed countries the vaccine has been shown to confer protection for at least three years, this has not been the case for children in developing countries. A study published in *Vaccine* in 2017 notes that, while the risk from rotavirus is greater in younger children, observations from poorer countries "raise concern that waning immunity may leave vaccinated children vulnerable to rotavirus diarrhea morbidity and mortality in the second year of life and beyond."[37]

As noted in a study published in the *Journal of the Royal Society Interface*, the immunity conferred by vaccination is like natural immunity in that "vaccines do not protect against infection but do protect against disease". However, while a child's first infection with rotavirus does not provide long-lasting protection against future infection, a second infection does confer an immunity "that protects completely against subsequent moderate-to-severe diarrhoea".

Frequent reexposures to rotavirus serve to maintain that protective natural immunity indefinitely, helping to ensure that future infections remain mild or asymptomatic. Ironically, the study concluded that "the success of rotavirus vaccine at an individual and population level" was likely dependent upon "the regular re-exposure of vaccine recipients to asymptomatic infection to maintain immunity, at least in the early years."[38]

The 2017 *Vaccine* paper proposed investigating the option of adding a third "booster" dose of rotavirus vaccine in developing countries to reduce mortality resulting from the waning of vaccine-conferred immunity.[39]

A study published in *Lancet Infectious Diseases* in July 2019 also examined the phenomenon of vaccine-conferred immunity waning more rapidly in resource-poor, high-mortality settings compared to high-income, low-mortality settings. A pivotal study in Mexico, a medium-mortality setting, found that "two previous infections (asymptomatic or symptomatic) conferred 100% protection against subsequent moderate or severe rotavirus gastroenteritis." Yet another pivotal study in India, a high-mortality setting, found that "the equivalent protection was 57%", so it is to be expected that vaccine efficacy would be lower in such settings.[40]

However, the study further observed, in addition to the more rapid waning of vaccine-induced antibodies in low-income settings, some of the decrease in estimated efficacy "could be explained by a higher incidence of natural asymptomatic and mild infections (and thus preferential immune boosting) among unvaccinated controls compared with vaccine recipients. *In these circumstances the risk of severe rotavirus gastroenteritis in vaccine recipients would gradually converge with, and might exceed, the risk in unvaccinated controls over time.*" (Emphasis added.)

Consistent with that hypothesis, the authors' analysis of the schedule for rotavirus vaccination in Indonesia "suggested a positive protective effect of the vaccine in the first 18 months of follow-up, but extrapolation of the curves suggested a negative effect thereafter." While "live oral rotavirus vaccines are still likely to provide substantial benefit" since most disease morbidity and mortality occur in children under two years old, as mass vaccination shifts the age of symptomatic infection to older children, "the need for more durable rotavirus vaccines might become more pressing."[41]

In addition to waning of vaccine-conferred immunity, shedding of vaccine-strain virus can also occur. A case report published in *Pediatrics* in 2010 documented the first known transmission from a vaccinated child to an unvaccinated sibling, which resulted in the unvaccinated sibling receiving emergency department care for rotavirus gastroenteritis.[42] A randomized placebo-controlled study published in *Vaccine* in 2011 examined this question in twins by giving one sibling in each pair the vaccine and the other a placebo. It found that, while not associated with symptomatic gastroenteritis, vaccinated infants transmitted vaccine-strain virus to their sibling 18.8 percent of the time.[43]

A study published in *Vaccine* in 2015 found the rotavirus vaccines used in the United States today to be associated with a small but statistically significant increased risk of intussusception, a painful and potentially fatal medical emergency in which the intestine telescopes in on itself, three to seven days after vaccination.[44]

This is not an entirely unsurprising finding since, as already discussed, the first rotavirus vaccine approved by the FDA and recommended for routine use in infants by the CDC was withdrawn from the market after it was found to be causing intussusception.

In addition to the board *falsely* claiming that rotavirus is "fully vaccine-preventable", Dr. Thomas says that the twins' parents had on multiple occasions declined all vaccines. They signed declination forms on August 21, 2018; October 16, 2018; December 28, 2018; April 15, 2019; June 23, 2019; September 11, 2019; and December 4, 2019. He says that the parents told him they had also declined all vaccines at the hospital where the twins were born and where they were treated for rotavirus at ten months of age.

The board's statement about the lack of chronic medical conditions that would "justify" their declination, Dr. Thomas observes, completely misses the point that the family was exercising their right to informed consent.

The reason the parents did not vaccinate, Thomas also explained, is "because they have a family history of severe autism." They had decided against vaccinations before ever coming into Thomas's practice. As he explained:

I actually had not seen those twins for their well-baby visits, but, never-theless, I got named as the one guilty for not getting them to vaccinate. They've signed vaccine refusal forms, and this comes back to the fact that where the board is mistaken and misguided is thinking that I'm push-ing this family not to vaccinate. It's actually the other way around. They come in not wanting to vaccinate. Sometimes, by going through informed consent, some families will actually give a vaccine they weren't planning to give.

He also suggested that if the mother told staff at the hospital that she thought that the twins were vaccinated, it was probably because she was under duress and sought to avoid confrontation about their decision not to vaccinate with other doctors who are not as respectful of their right not to do so. Another possibility, he noted, is that she never made such a statement.

He also said that the parents informed him of their belief that their twins probably were infected with rotavirus by a vaccinated neighbor child.

Additionally, he had been informed by the parents that their case might be used against him by the medical board. "While they were in the hospital," Thomas said, "they overheard the infectious disease doctor—after her rotation in the room, standing outside the room—tell her little group of students and medical students, 'I'm gonna turn that doctor in. Doesn't he know there's a vaccine for rotavirus?'"

"Of course," Thomas added, "the board won't tell you who initiated any complaint."

Testing for Measles Antibody Titers

In addition to the eight patient cases cited to support its accusations, the medical board faulted Dr. Thomas for ordering tests for 905 patients to determine blood antibody levels, or "titers," for measles, mumps, and rubella. The board stated that, "[e]xcept for rare cases of suspected immune deficiency, there is no clinical indication for assessment of anti-body titers. The ordering of unnecessary testing is a violation of ORS 677.190(1)(a) unprofessional or dishonorable conduct, as defined in ORS 677.188(4)(c) willful and repeated ordering or performance of unnecessary laboratory tests."[45]

In the case of 122 patients, tests indicated "an inadequate response to the mumps vaccines", and thirty-two of those "received the appropriate second dose of mumps vaccine." The board asserted that the other ninety should have received the second dose, as well, stating that, "[r]egardless of antibody titers, the standard of care requires a second dose of the recommended MMR vaccination." The board accused Thomas of having "failed to ensure these patients were given the required second dose of MMR as soon as he obtained the test results. Knowingly leaving these children inadequately protected against a preventable, potentially debilitating illness constitutes 90 acts of gross and repeated negligence" and "constitutes unprofessional or dishonorable conduct" that "does or might constitute a danger to the health or safety of a patient or the public."

However, if performing unnecessary medical interventions is an offense for which physicians should lose their licenses, then it is every other doctor who administers the second dose of the MMR vaccine *without* first ordering an antibody test who is guilty of unprofessional conduct constituting a danger to public health.

The board's suspension order fails to acknowledge the whole rationale for testing for antibodies before administering the second dose, which is precisely to *avoid* placing children at risk of harm from an *unnecessary* vaccination.

The fact that the second dose of MMR vaccine is *unnecessary* for *most* children is not controversial. As the CDC itself explains, "Approximately 90%–95% of recipients of a single dose" of the MMR vaccine "develop protective antibody within 2 weeks of the dose. However, because a limited proportion of recipients (≤5%) of MMR vaccine fail to respond to one dose, a second dose is recommended to provide another opportunity to develop immunity."[46]

In other words, for *most* children who get the MMR vaccine, the second dose is *unnecessary*, but the CDC recommends all children receive the second dose *anyway* rather than doing antibody testing to identify the minority who experience vaccine failure. (A certain proportion of non-responders to the first dose will also fail to respond to the second dose.)

Hence, it is the CDC itself that is responsible for establishing as "standard of care" a medical procedure that for *most* children poses *an unnecessary risk of harm*.

The board's accusation is even more ludicrous given the fact that Oregon law only requires *one* dose of *mumps* vaccine, and it *specifically allows for the use of antibody testing as evidence of immunity in lieu of evidence of vaccination.*

At the time of this writing, on the Oregon government's website, the Oregon Health Authority's page titled "Exemptions and Immunity" states that parents who do not want their children to be vaccinated can claim an exemption *or* "show immunity because of having had a disease *or with a blood test.*" (Emphasis added.)

It specifically states that a person who can show evidence of immunity does not need to provide evidence of vaccination and that "[i]mmunity documentation is acceptable for history of disease or positive titer (blood test) for hepatitis B, hepatitis A, Hib, MMR or varicella."[47]

Under Oregon law, the school attendance requirement is for *one* dose for the mumps and rubella portions of the MMR vaccine. It requires two doses only for the measles component.[48] Consequently, antibody tests indicating a failed response to the mumps portion of the vaccine are completely irrelevant. Parents are not required to get their children a second dose for *mumps*, and Dr. Thomas is certainly not required under the law to *force* parents to do so.

Since it is a combination vaccine, a second dose for measles also means a second dose for mumps and rubella, but the law also explicitly allows for the use of antibody tests as evidence of immunity *in lieu of the second dose*. It states that to continue attendance at school, a child must be up to date with vaccinations, have an exemption, *or* have "immunity documentation".[49]

The requirement for vaccination may legally be satisfied by a physician certifying "a disease history", meaning that the child has acquired natural immunity through infection, *or* evidence of immunity in the form of "a documented immune titer". The law specifies that for the MMR vaccine, "a documented immune titer" certified by a physician "satisfies the immunization requirements".[50]

Apart from the fact that the board accused Dr. Thomas of "unprofessional conduct" *for doing something explicitly provided for under Oregon law*, the bottom line is that his patients' parents had a *right* to request antibody testing and a *right* to decline the second dose of MMR vaccine *regardless* of whether their child experienced vaccine failure with the first dose. Dr. Thomas had both an *ethical* and a *legal obligation* to respect parents' decisions to exercise that right.

If the law in Oregon was being upheld to prevent doctors from ordering *unnecessary* procedures that *carry a risk of harm*, the Oregon Medical Board would be going after doctors who refuse parents' requests for an antibody test and insist that their children receive the second dose of the MMR vaccine.

Dr. Paul's Summation of the Medical Board's Allegations

Paul Thomas rejects the board's accusation that he tries to pressure parents one way or the other with respect to vaccination. He sees it as his duty to properly *inform* so that individuals can make their own decision.

"Almost all of their complaints are mistaken complaints in how they are interpreting what happens with informed consent," he said. In each of his examine rooms, on the wall across from or right next to where the parents sit is the CDC's schedule, and he goes through it with them during well-visits.

He noted that few parents who come to his practice decide to strictly comply with the CDC's schedule. This may be partly because, unlike other pediatricians, he doesn't push the CDC schedule on their children, which he views as unethical behavior and true bullying. However, it is also a result of his reputation in the community. "They are specifically coming to my office," he said, "because they want informed consent."

His published data show that he has had 561 patients born into his practice who were completely unvaccinated. The parents of these patients made this decision not because he pressured them but because "nobody on this Earth is going to convince them to do it."

So, you know," he added, "it's interesting that they're going to target me because these people are choosing their legal right not to vaccinate."

What Dr. Paul's Patient Data Tell Us about the Health of Unvaccinated Children

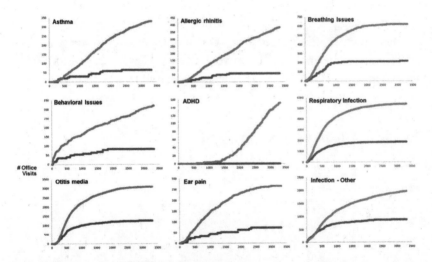

Dr. Paul Thomas's published data indicate that his completely unvaccinated patients are the healthiest children in his practice.

Dr. Thomas obtained Institutional Review Board approval to use his clinic's data for research purposes on May 7, 2019. The analyses of the deidentified data were done by Dr. James Lyons-Weiler. Their study, titled "Relative Incidence of Office Visits and Cumulative Rates of Billed Diagnoses Along the Axis of Vaccination," was published in the

International Journal of Environmental Research and Public Health on November 22, 2020.

In the paper's introduction, they noted the lack of studies comparing long-term health outcomes between vaccinated and completely unvaccinated children. A typical vaccine safety study employs "an '*N* vs. *N* + 1' design of analysis, meaning they compare fully vaccinated children with fully vaccinated children missing only one vaccine."[1] A few independent studies had been done looking at completely unvaccinated children, such as by Mawson et al. in 2017 and Hooker and Miller in 2020.

The study population using Dr. Thomas's clinical data was limited to those born into the practice. This avoided confounding with health outcomes related to the fact that children would not have been vaccinated according to the vaccine-friendly plan's standard of individualized care and informed consent. It also avoided confounding due to health-care-seeking behaviors that might differ between practices, such as parents being more hesitant to take their child in due to the anxiety caused by not wanting to be lectured about their vaccination choices.

The patients' ages ranged from two months to 10.4 years, with high variability in vaccination. There were 2,763 patients who were variably vaccinated and 561 who were totally unvaccinated:

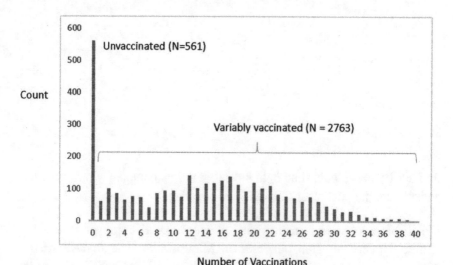

Figure 2 in the study shows the distribution of vaccination across the patient cohort.

They noted that "healthy user bias" was a confounding factor of special concern for vaccine safety studies, since parents whose children are predisposed to certain diseases or disorders may choose not to vaccinate precisely because they notice early symptoms or because an older sibling who'd been vaccinated had been diagnosed with a chronic health condition, resulting in children at higher risk of being diagnosed with the condition being disproportionately pooled into the "unvaccinated" group.

If their findings were explainable by "healthy user bias" as it has been described, then we would expect to see more illness in the unvaccinated. They found just the opposite despite observing "the potential signal of informed avoidance of vaccine injury with informed consent and without coercion".

That signal was evident in their finding that there was a family history of autoimmunity with 31 percent of the unvaccinated compared to 25.16 percent of the variably vaccinated. They suggested that this "likely reflects the net effects of decisions between the patient/doctor dyad in determining risk of long-term poor outcomes sometimes associated with vaccination."

Another confounding factor they accounted for was the relationship between the number of vaccines received and age. Naturally, older children would tend to have had more vaccines than younger children. To avoid comparing vaccinated children with long-term care in Dr. Thomas's practice and unvaccinated children with short-term care, they matched patients between the two groups according to "days of care" in the practice. Since all patients were born into the practice, this correlated with age. Matching patients to days of care also served to protect against finding different health outcomes due to different healthcare-seeking behavior.

As they explained:

> Typical retrospective analyses of association of outcomes and vaccine exposure rely on incidence of conditions, which is the percentage of a group with a particular diagnosis of interest. This is the equivalent of "at least one billed office visit", which is a specific form of "at least n office visits" related to a diagnosis. Use of incidence-only is therefore an arbitrary decision on data representation. We generalized the approach by considering the incidence of office visits over each patients' record related to diagnosis.[2]

Their study was not a comparison of children fully vaccinated according to the CDC's schedule and unvaccinated children due to the approach taken by Dr. Thomas of providing individualized care and respecting informed consent. These are key elements of his vaccine-friendly plan, which also aims to space out aluminum-containing vaccines and to choose vaccines without aluminum if available. The net effect of this approach on aluminum accumulation in children was described in their prior study, published in the *Journal of Trace Elements in Medicine and Biology* in December 2019.

Compared to children following the CDC schedule, the most highly vaccinated patients in Thomas's practice received fourteen fewer vaccines by age two, four fewer additional vaccines by age five, and six fewer additional vaccines by age ten. Consequently, children following the CDC schedule would have received twenty-four additional doses compared to the most highly vaccinated patients in Thomas's practice.

To further control for differences in healthcare-seeking behavior between vaccinated and unvaccinated patients, they also looked at incidence of fever and well-child visits. Since fever is a known adverse event associated with vaccination, it was expected that the unvaccinated would

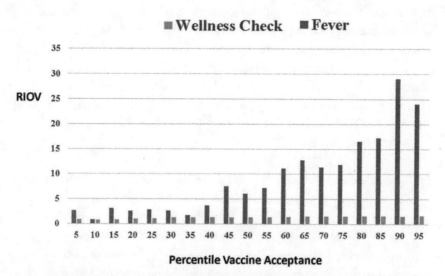

Figure 3 in the study shows the RIOV percentile for fever and well-child visits, with RIOV representing the total number of billed office visits per condition per group, which reflects the total disease burden in that study population.

have fewer visits for fever. If differences in health outcomes were explainable by parents of unvaccinated children simply choosing not to go in to see their pediatrician, it would also be expected that these patients would have fewer well-child visits.

As expected, they found that children who received more vaccines had a higher relative incidence of office visits (RIOV) for fever than children who received none. However, there was a stable trend for relative incidence of well-child visits, indicating that differences in healthcare-seeking behavior did not account for the lower incidence of fever in children who received fewer or no vaccines.

In one analysis, they used the typical method of calculating an odds ratio and relative risk comparing incidence of diagnoses between vaccinated and unvaccinated children.[3] Additionally, they analyzed the data using their new method of comparing relative incidence of office visits. Using both measures, they showed a higher incidence of diagnoses among

Table 5. Analysis 4: DOC-matched incidence analysis.

Outcome	OR	RR	95% CI	ARD	Significance
Fever	3.88	3.66	2.02/2.75	0.057	+,+
Ear Pain	1.559	1.57	0.723/0.966	0.01	−,−
Otitis media	1.551	1.4	1.17/1.22	0.078	+,+
Otitis externa	2.01	1.996	0.602	1	+,+
Conjunctivitis	1.323	1.273	0.942/1.05	0.033	−,+
Eye Disorders—Other	1.25	1.24	0.729/0.879	0.011	−,−
Ear Disorders	1.29	1.28	0.476/0.671	0.003	−,−
Asthma	1.224	1.22	0.503/0.679	0.003	−,−
Allergic Rhinitis	1.452	1.44	0.615/0.842	0.007	−,−
Sinusitis	1.2	1.2	0.364/0.540	0.008	−,−
Breathing Issues	1.614	1.549	1.504/1.217	0.037	+,+
Anemia	3.216	2.865	2.098/2.368	0.103	+,+
Eczema	2.822	2.682	1.57/2.01	0.047	+,+
Urticaria	1	1	0.471/0.595	0	−,−
Dermatitis	0.884	0.898	1.27/1.13	−0.012	+,+
Behavioral Issues	2.13	2.067	1.11/1.45	0.0266	+,+
Gastroenteritis	2.785	2.572	1.74/2.054	0.073	+,+
Weight/Eating Disorders	1.915	1.721	1.386/1.47	0.089	+,+
Allergy—Food	0.498	0.499	5.51/3.53	−0.001	−,−
Seizure	1.756	1.746	0.511/0.836	0.0053	−,−
Infection—Respiratory	1.716	1.365	1.351/1.255	0.131	+,+
Pain	1.274	1.255	0.783/0.927	0.014	−,−

The symbols "+, −" denote the significance of the relevant (upper or lower) 95% CI analysis for OR and RR.

Table 5 of the study shows the DOC-matched incidence of diagnoses analysis with odds ratio (OR) and relative risk (RR) presented for diagnosed condition.

the vaccinated children, with the signal being more pronounced when measuring RIOV.

This result was largely to be expected since the number of vaccines administered correlates with age. After controlling for this by matching unvaccinated and vaccinated patients for days of care (DOC), "many of the conditions for which associations were found in the RIOV analysis were found to be undetectable" when calculating the odds ratio for incidence of diagnosis. Conditions for which a significant association remained included fever, otitis media, otitis externa, breathing issues, anemia, eczema, dermatitis, behavioral issues, gastroenteritis, weight or eating disorders, and respiratory infection.

The RIOV was also reduced in the DOC-matched analysis, but "the significance of an increased proportion of cases in the vaccinated individuals compared to unvaccinated individuals remains for most outcomes." Conditions for which a statistically significant association remained

Table 3. RIOV analysis of outcomes of the vaccinated vs. unvaccinated groups, matched for Days of Care (DOC) matched comparison (N1 = 561 and N2 = 561).

Condition	Vaxxed	Unvaxxed	RIOV	95% CI	Z	P(Z)
					Test of Proportions	
Fever	78	17	4.596	4.412	6.547	<0.00001
"Well Child" Visit	5204	4989	1.045	1.041	2.156	0.0307
Ear Pain	18	16	1.127	1.022	0.354	0.726
Otitis media	355	216	1.646	1.001	8.312	<0.00001
Conjunctivitis	113	87	1.301	1.023	2.042	0.04136
Eye Disorders—Other	38	31	1.228	1.076	0.877	0.3788
Asthma	20	13	1.541	1.437	1.317	0.186
Allergic Rhinitis	21	12	1.753	1.649	1.600	0.1096
Sinusitis	6	5	1.202	1.143	0.306	0.756
Breathing Issues	75	44	1.708	1.502	3.015	0.00252
Anemia	130	36	3.618	3.361	7.912	<0.00001
Eczema	64	23	2.788	2.613	4.581	<0.00001
Urticaria	14	17	0.825	0.925	−0.541	0.5892
Dermatitis	86	105	0.821	1.090	−1.459	0.1443
Behavioral Issues	54	17	3.182	3.026	4.452	<0.00001
Gastroenteritis	89	30	2.972	2.763	5.728	<0.00001
Weight/Eating Disorders	147	92	1.601	1.288	4.023	<0.00001
Seizure	10	8	0.798	0.067	0.874	0.6312
Respiratory Infection	703	382	2.682	1.134	51.85	<0.00001

The calculation of Z for "Well Child" visits compared the proportion of number of office visits per group to the total number of days of care (length of time in practice; per group: vaccinated = 416,101, unvaccinated 416,056) in this DOC-matched analysis.

Table 3 of the study shows the DOC-matched relative incidence of office visits (RIOV) with an RIOV greater than one indicating higher incidence among the vaccinated patients.

included fever, otitis media, conjunctivitis, breathing issues, anemia, eczema, behavioral issues, gastroenteritis, weight or eating disorders, and respiratory infection.

In another analysis, they compared cumulative office visits per condition for vaccinated and unvaccinated patients over time. Since there were fewer unvaccinated patients in the study population, the cumulative office visits curve for the unvaccinated was multiplied by 4.9 to adjust for the office visits expected if the number of unvaccinated patients was equal to the number of vaccinated. This made the two curves directly comparable in scale.

The resulting graphs are striking, showing that unvaccinated patients had significantly less cumulative office visits for asthma, allergic rhinitis, eczema, dermatitis, urticaria, breathing issues, anemia, respiratory infections, other infections, otitis media, behavioral issues, and ADHD.

A further analysis showed that RIOV is a more statistically powerful measure than incidence of diagnosis. As they explained, "Office visits carry more information than diagnoses; specifically, measures based on the number of office visits will carry information on severity in addition to the number of yes/no ever-diagnoses." The reduced statistical power of odds ratios on incidence of diagnoses relative to RIOV analysis "may help explain the failure of many prior studies to detect an association between exposure to vaccines and adverse health effects."

Yet another analysis looked at rates of diagnoses for diseases that CDC-recommended vaccines are intended to protect against. They found a total of forty-one such diagnoses: twenty-nine for varicella (or chicken pox), ten for pertussis, and two for rotavirus. The respective numbers of diagnoses for the unvaccinated group were twenty-three, nine, and two. These numbers indicated that 17.2 children born into Dr. Thomas's practice required vaccination for one child to receive the benefit of protection against a vaccine-targeted disease.[4]

To put it another way, for every seventeen children vaccinated, sixteen received no benefit from having undergone that risk-carrying pharmaceutical intervention. Importantly, there were zero deaths in Dr. Thomas's practice from any disease for which the CDC recommends vaccination.

There were not enough patients in Dr. Thomas's practice with diagnosed neurodevelopmental conditions to be able to draw any

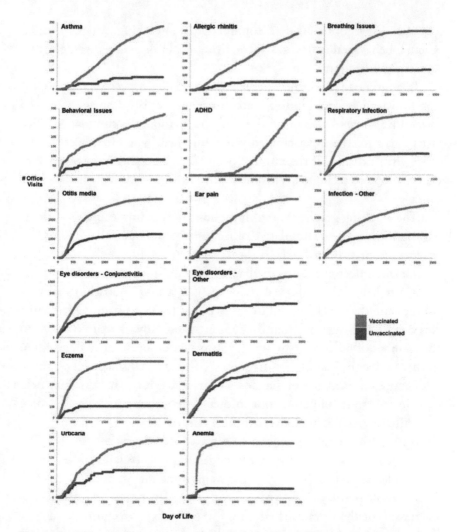

Figure 5 of the study compares cumulative office visits per condition in the vaccinated (lighter) with unvaccinated (darker) patients over time (days of life).

meaningful conclusions by including this category in their analyses comparing unvaccinated with variably vaccinated children, but the fact that there were low rates of such conditions is by itself remarkable.

According to the CDC, the national prevalence of autism is one in fifty-four children.[5] This reflects the rate of autism in a highly vaccinated population. By comparison, the rate of autism among patients born into

Dr. Thomas's practice—a population that in CDC parlance is heavily "undervaccinated"—was one in 277. That is, the rate of autism in their study population was one-fifth that of the US national rate.

Just as remarkably, there were zero unvaccinated patients in the study population with ADHD compared to 5.3 percent of the variably vaccinated.[6] That rate in turn compares with the US national rate, according to the CDC, of 9.4 percent.[7]

It is difficult to see how the findings of their study could be attributed to differences in healthcare-seeking behavior or lifestyle choices *separate* from the parental choice not to vaccinate. As Lyons-Weiler and Thomas remark, if their findings are explainable by different lifestyle choices, "then it would be objective to conclude that everyone should adopt the lifestyle followed by the unvaccinated if they want healthier children. That lifestyle choice includes, for many families, avoiding some or all vaccines, and thus, the lifestyle choice concern is inextricably linked to vaccine exposure."

They also noted that their findings were not generalizable to other pediatric practices or the general US childhood population due to Dr. Thomas's unique approach of individualized care and respect for informed consent, in keeping with the principles of his vaccine-friendly plan.

Further research should be done, they suggested, using data from other pediatric practices, and researchers should focus on the relative incidence of billed office visits due to the increased statistical power inherent in using a measure reflecting disease severity compared with the "binary yes/no incidence of diagnoses."

As they summarized their findings, "We could detect no widespread negative health effects in the unvaccinated other than the rare but significant vaccine-targeted diagnoses. We can conclude that the unvaccinated children in this practice are not, overall, less healthy than the vaccinated and that indeed the vaccinated children appear to be significantly less healthy than the unvaccinated."[8]

Conclusion

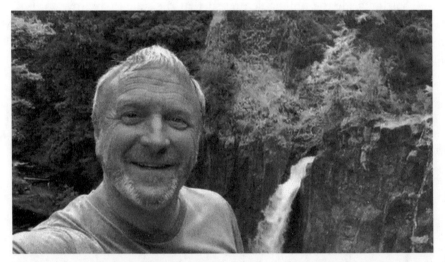

Paul Thomas hiking at Drift Creek Falls, Oregon, from a video he shot encouraging people to get out in nature *(photo courtesy of Paul Thomas)*

The Oregon state government would like us to believe that Dr. Paul Thomas and any other physicians who do not maintain a high vaccination rate in their pediatric practice represent a danger to society. The reality is that the threat to public health in this regard is coming from government officials like those on the Oregon Medical Board who advocate mass vaccination as a one-size-fits-all solution to infectious disease and are intent on waging an all-out assault on our right to informed consent.

What science tells us is not that all vaccines are equally "safe and effective" for everyone, but that a risk-benefit analysis must be done for each vaccine *and every individual.* That is precisely the approach Dr. Thomas has taken in his practice, *in accordance with the requirement under Oregon law that he obtain informed consent*, yet he is being punished for it.

The Oregon Medical Board has tried to conceal the true reason for its suspension of Dr. Thomas's license by accusing him of pressuring patients into choosing *not* to receive vaccines according to the CDC's recommendations, but it is patently obvious that the state has no problem whatsoever with bullying physicians, such as those who kick patients out of their practice if they do not strictly comply with the CDC schedule.

Indeed, the clear message delivered by the suspension order is that doctors *must* bully their patients into accepting vaccinations *or risk losing their license to practice medicine*.

Setting aside the untenable pretext that the state disapproves of bullying physicians, it also becomes manifestly obvious that the true reason why Dr. Thomas was stripped of his license is that he respects parents' right to informed consent for vaccinations, which is a standard of care that is incompatible with the state government's myopic approach.

It is also instructive that the Oregon Medical Board saw fit to have an "emergency" meeting to suspend Dr. Thomas's license just days after he published a *requested* peer-reviewed study showing that his respect for informed consent is *not* risking the health and lives of his pediatric patients, but, on the contrary, is associated with enviable health outcomes.

Preventing Dr. Thomas from helping his pediatric patients is not the only problem that the medical board has created. In addition to being a pediatrician, Thomas is also an addiction specialist and coauthor with Dr. Jennifer Margulis of the book *The Addiction Spectrum*. The medical board's decision has also stopped him from being able to help teens and young adults get off opiate drugs, with the opioid epidemic being another crisis that the medical establishment has been largely responsible for creating.[1]

Evidently, when the board requested Dr. Thomas to produce peer-reviewed data supporting the approach espoused in his vaccine-friendly plan, it was expected that he would not be able to do so. Of course, the Oregon Medical Board cannot produce any studies showing that health outcomes are better for children vaccinated according to the CDC's schedule than for completely unvaccinated children because, as the Institute of Medicine has observed, such studies do not exist.

But setting aside the sheer hypocrisy, the fact that he defied their expectation and produced the data *only to have his license emergently suspended as a result* illustrates how the board remains ignorantly fixated on the policy agenda of maintaining high vaccination rates *rather than focusing on health outcomes.*

The state's rejection of the right to informed consent is evident not only in its suspension of Dr. Thomas, but also in its "education" module that parents must endure if they wish to obtain a so-called "nonmedical" exemption but cannot find a doctor like Paul Thomas who will write one for them. Far from providing them with the knowledge they need to be able to make an informed choice, the videos insult parents' intelligence and *misinform* them for the purpose of persuasion. It is patently intended not to educate, but to manufacture consent for state policy.

Indeed, the state's goal of achieving high vaccination rates is *fundamentally incompatible with the goal of educating people to be able to make their own informed choice.* The state simply wants people to unquestioningly obey. This explains why they have gone after Dr. Paul Thomas for enabling parents to exercise their right to decline vaccinations. In essence, the state, in addition to coercing parents to vaccinate, is now following California's lead by also coercing doctors to do the same.

It is also not a coincidence that shortly after the medical board issued its "emergency" suspension order, a bill was introduced into the Oregon Senate that, in the words of the legislative summary, "[r]emoves ability of parent to decline required immunizations against restrictable diseases on behalf of child for reason other than child's indicated medical diagnosis."

The bill further "[d]irects boards that regulate certain licensed health care practitioners to review documents completed by licensed health care practitioners granting exemptions from immunization requirements because of indicated medical diagnosis."[2]

In other words, if this piece of legislation, Senate Bill 254, becomes law, the state of Oregon will have adopted California Senator Richard Pan's view that exempting children from state-mandated vaccines is not the practice of medicine, *but an administrative function performed by physicians in service to the state.* This is a totally unacceptable and dangerous intervention by government bureaucrats into the doctor-patient relationship.

As the study by Dr. Lyons-Weiler and Dr. Thomas shows, the completely unvaccinated children in the latter's practice are not unhealthier than those who have been variably vaccinated. On the contrary, the data strongly suggest that they are the healthiest children in his practice, with significantly less incidence of diagnoses and fewer office visits for a broad range of chronic illnesses.

If we are to have a hope of addressing the epidemic of chronic illnesses among the childhood population, a chief obstacle that *must* be overcome is the medical establishment's government-legislated approach of coercing people into accepting pharmaceutical interventions. The policy goal of achieving high vaccination rates *must no longer supersede the goal of achieving a healthy childhood population.*

Just as when he refused to raise the flag of an apartheid regime as a child growing up in Africa, Dr. Thomas has taken a courageous stand against the government and the corrupt medical establishment in the United States. He knew when he published his book *The Vaccine-Friendly Plan* that he was risking his career, but he did so anyway because he could not in good conscience continue practicing medicine in blind obedience to institutions that have proven themselves over and over to be completely unworthy of our trust.

To arrive at that place, he had to undergo his own journey of awakening. Unfortunately, too few doctors seem willing to consider the possibility that something they are doing with the intent of helping children is instead causing harm. Dr. Thomas had to overcome that confirmation bias and face that realization, which ultimately caused him to leave his private group practice and open Integrative Pediatrics. The health outcomes he has achieved as a result are now documented in a peer-reviewed study that the Oregon Medical Board clearly does not care to consider.

The problem is not that there are too many physicians like Dr. Paul Thomas out there, *but that there are far too few.* By suspending his license essentially for practicing informed consent, the government of Oregon has not only gone after one doctor *but effectively declared war on the right of parents everywhere to make informed choices about how best to achieve good health for their children.*

As a simple logical truism, government bureaucrats do not have the requisite knowledge *of the individual child* to be able to conduct a meaningful risk-benefit analysis on the child's behalf. *Only* the parents working in consultation with their child's physician have that essential knowledge. We must not allow government to insert itself even further into that doctor-patient relationship, and the extent to which government has already done so must be reversed.

The increasingly authoritarian government policies related to the practice of vaccination represent an existential threat to both our health and our liberty. Those who value both must take a stand now against abusive government policies for the sake of future generations of humanity.

Afterword

After this book was written, on June 3, 2021, the Oregon Medical Board conditionally withdrew its Order of Emergency Suspension against Dr. Paul Thomas. While this may rightly be viewed as a victory by the health freedom movement, the board's investigation into his practice is ongoing, and Dr. Thomas still faces an immense legal battle. In the meantime, the board is still inserting itself into his doctor-patient relationship and restricting his ability to practice as he and his patients deem fit. Furthermore, his battle represents just one of many fronts in the ongoing war against our right to informed consent, which now includes efforts to pressure people into accepting experimental COVID-19 vaccines (which at this time of writing have not received FDA approval, and for which phase three clinical trials are ongoing). Readers wishing to stand with Dr. Thomas and support his courageous efforts to fight on all our behalf can learn more at www.paulthomasmd.com.

About the Author

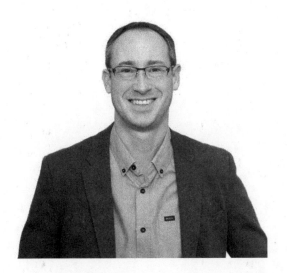

Jeremy R. Hammond is an independent journalist, political analyst, and author. He has written about a wide variety of topics, including US foreign policy, economic policy, and public vaccine policy, always with a particular focus on exposing dangerous government and media propaganda intended to manufacture public consent for harmful policies. His other books include *Obstacle to Peace: The US Role in the Israeli-Palestinian Conflict* and *Ron Paul vs. Paul Krugman: Austrian vs. Keynesian Economics in the Financial Crisis*. Find his work and sign up for his newsletter at JeremyRHammond.com.

Acknowledgments: I would like to thank Dr. James Lyons-Weiler for alerting me to the publication of the study "Relative Incidence of Office Visits and Cumulative Rates of Billed Diagnoses Along the Axis of Vaccination" and the Oregon Medical Board's subsequent "emergency" order suspending Dr. Paul Thomas's license. Dr. Lyons-Weiler also connected me directly with Dr. Thomas, including arranging for an online interview. This article benefited from questions asked during that interview by Alix Mayer from Children's Health Defense. I thank Dr. Thomas for giving me his time and answering my many questions both during our interview and in numerous follow-up emails.

Conflicts of Interest: I received no fee, wage, salary, commission, grant, or other form of payment to write the published article from which this book has been adapted. This work was funded by donations I regularly receive from readers who value my independent journalism. I did mention on several occasions in my newsletters that I was working on an article about the Oregon Medical Board's suspension of Dr. Paul Thomas's license, but none of my supporting readers had any involvement beyond making a financial contribution to support my work generally, with or without the knowledge that I was even working on the article. I have one conflict of interest to declare: *I am a father.*

Notes

Introduction

1   Oregon Medical Board, "In the Matter of Paul Norman Thomas, MD, License No. MD15689: Order of Emergency Suspension," State of Oregon, December 3, 2020, https://omb.oregon.gov/Clients/ORMB/OrderDocuments/e579dd35-7e1b-471f -a69a-3a800317ed4c.pdf.

2   In my own case, our son's pediatrician told us during an early well-child visit that Wakefield was serving time in prison for what he'd done, which I knew was untrue. This attempt to persuade us into compliance consequently served only to reaffirm our conviction that we shouldn't assume doctors are trustworthy and should rather do our own research, think for ourselves, and trust our own judgment.

3   I, too, have experienced rifts within my family over this issue, and, naturally, as someone who has for years been publicly criticizing public vaccine policy, I have experienced countless personal attacks on my character.

4   My wife and I have likewise experienced this, very recently, due to a policy change at our son's pediatric practice. On May 5, 2021, we were given an ultimatum by one of the doctors there to either vaccinate him according to the AAP's recommendations (synonymous with the CDC's recommendations) or never come back. We declined the unnecessary and risk-carrying pharmaceutical products and so were expelled. Several years prior, we were also expelled from the practice of the only pediatric dentist in town because we persistently declined fluoride treatment. She lied on his dental record, stating that he had several cavities. He was three then. We showed his X-rays to another dentist whom we trusted, and he agreed with us that it showed no cavities, which he also confirmed with an oral examination. We continued taking our son to biannual cleanings at another local clinic, where dentists also confirmed for years after that he had no cavities. I filed a complaint with the state licensing board, but the board sided with her, thereby granting its approval of her expelling my son from her practice on account of our exercising our right to informed consent. This experience reflects that of many parents with their pediatrician over vaccination choices.

5   James Lyons-Weiler and Paul Thomas, "Relative Incidence of Office Visits and Cumulative Rates of Billed Diagnoses Along the Axis of Vaccination," *International Journal of Environmental Research and Public Health*, November 22, 2020, https://doi .org/10.3390/ijerph17228674.

6   Oregon Medical Board, "Order of Emergency Suspension."

The Path of a Pro-Vaccine Pediatrician

1   David Mark, photo of the Dartmouth College campus library building, Pixabay, accessed May 1, 2021, https://pixabay.com/photos/dartmouth-college-campus-school -292587/. Licensed under Pixabay License, https://pixabay.com/service/license/.

2   Richard Smith, "Thoughts for new medical students at a new medical school," *BMJ*, December 20, 2003, https://www.ncbi.nlm.nih.gov/pmc/articles/PMC300793/.

The Proven Untrustworthiness of Public Health Officials

1   Daniel Mayer, photo of the entrance to the headquarters of the Centers for Disease Control and Prevention, taken April 24, 2011, available from Wikimedia Commons, accessed May 1, 2021, https://commons.wikimedia.org/wiki/File:Centers_for _Disease_Control_and_Prevention_-_Main_entrance.JPG. Licensed under Creative Commons Attribution-ShareAlike 3.0 Unported (CC BY-SA 3.0), https:// creativecommons.org/licenses/by-sa/3.0/deed.en.

2   Centers for Disease Control and Prevention, "Polio Disease–Questions and Answers," *CDC.gov*, updated August 11, 2014; archived at https://web.archive.org /web/20150103130229/https://www.cdc.gov/vaccines/vpd-vac/polio/dis-faqs.htm.

3   Food and Drug Administration, "Additional Standards for Viral Vaccines; Poliovirus Vaccine, Live, Oral," Federal Register, Vol. 49, No. 107, June 1, 1984, https://www .govinfo.gov/app/details/FR-1984-06-01.

4   Jan Hoffman, "How Anti-Vaccine Sentiment Took Hold in the United States," *New York Times*, September 23, 2019, https://www.nytimes.com/2019/09/23/health/anti -vaccination-movement-us.html.

5   D L Miller et al., "Pertussis immunization and serious acute neurological illness in children," *British Medical Journal*, May 16, 1981, https://www.ncbi.nlm.nih.gov /pmc/articles/PMC1505512/.

6   R J Robinson, "The whooping-cough immmunisation controversy," *Archives of Disease in Childhood*, 1981, https://adc.bmj.com/content/archdischild/56/8/577.full.pdf; A R Hinman, "The pertussis vaccine controversy," *Public Health Reports*, May-June 1984, https://www.ncbi.nlm.nih.gov/pmc/articles/PMC1424579/.

7   Jenna Patterson et al., "Comparison of adverse events following immunisation with acellular and whole-cell pertussis vaccines: A systematic review," *Vaccine*, August 22, 2018, https://doi.org/10.1016/j.vaccine.2018.08.022.

8   Robert D. Grove and Alice M. Hetzel, *Vital Statistics Rates in the United States 1940–1960* (Washington, D.C.: US. Government Printing Office, 1968), https:// www.cdc.gov/nchs/data/vsus/vsrates1940_60.pdf. For further discussion, see: Jeremy R. Hammond, "Pertussis Vaccine Myth vs. Scientific Data," *JeremyRHammond. com*, September 9, 2020, https://www.jeremyrhammond.com/2020/09/09/pertussis -vaccine-myth-vs-scientific-data/.

9   Bernard Guyer et al., "Annual Summary of Vital Statistics: Trends in the Health of Americans During the 20th Century," *Pediatrics*, December 2000, https://doi .org/10.1542/peds.106.6.1307. See also: John B. McKinlay and Sonja M. McKinlay, "The Questionable Contribution of Medical Measures to the Decline of Mortality in the United States in the Twentieth Century," *The Milbank Quarterly*, 1977, https://

www.milbank.org/quarterly/articles/the-questionable-contribution-of-medical
-measures-to-the-decline-of-mortality-in-the-united-states-in-the-twentieth-century/.

10 Søren Wengel Mogensen et al., "The Introduction of Diphtheria-Tetanus-Pertussis and Oral Polio Vaccine Among Young Infants in an Urban African Community: A Natural Experiment," *EBioMedicine*, January 31, 2017, https://doi.org/10.1016/j.ebiom.2017.01.041.

11 Peter Aaby et al., "WHO's rollout of malaria vaccine in Africa: can safety questions be answered after only 24 months?" *The BMJ*, January 24, 2020, https://doi.org/10.1136/bmj.l6920.

12 Jeremy R. Hammond, "Is the Vaccine Injury Compensation Program Evidence of Vaccine Safety?" *JeremyRHammond.com*, July 1, 2019, https://www.jeremyrhammond.com/2019/07/01/is-the-vaccine-injury-compensation-program-evidence-of-vaccine-safety/.

13 Supreme Court of the United States, *Brueswitz et al. v. Wyeth LLC, FKA Wyeth, Inc., et al.*, February 22, 2011, https://www.supremecourt.gov/opinions/10pdf/09-152.pdf.

14 Lyn Redwood, "CDC Knew Its Vaccine Program Was Exposing Children to Dangerous Mercury Levels Since 1999," *Children's Health Defense*, January 20, 2017, https://childrenshealthdefense.org/news/cdc-knew-vaccine-program-exposing-children-dangerous-mercury-levels-since-1999/.

15 Leslie K. Ball, Robert Ball, and R. Douglas Pratt, "An Assessment of Thimerosal Use in Childhood Vaccines," *Pediatrics*, May 5, 2001, https://doi.org/10.1542/peds.107.5.1147. The FDA claimed that the mercury levels exceeded the guidelines set by the Environmental Protection Agency (EPA), but not those set by the Agency for Toxic Substances and Disease Registry (ATSDR) or the FDA itself. However, the FDA knew that was false. Its published results showed the levels based on the average exposure over the first six months of life, which is scientifically invalid, since, in real life, that is not how infants were exposed. Rather than very low-dose chronic exposure, they were exposed to repeated acute doses. An FDA consultant had shown that, looking at the instantaneous exposures from the schedule, the cumulative levels of mercury to which infants were exposed exceeded the FDA's own less stringent guidelines, as well. For further discussion and documentation, see: Jeremy R. Hammond, "The CDC's Criminal Recommendation for a Flu Shot During Pregnancy," *JeremyRHammond.com*, May 14, 2019, https://www.jeremyrhammond.com/2019/05/14/the-cdcs-criminal-recommendation-for-a-flu-shot-during-pregnancy/.

16 US House of Representatives, "Mercury in Medicine Report," Congressional Record Volume 149, Number 76, May 21, 2003, https://www.govinfo.gov/content/pkg/CREC-2003-05-21/html/CREC-2003-05-21-pt1-PgE1011-3.htm.

17 Redwood, "CDC Knew." See the email obtained through a Freedom of Information Act (FOIA) request from Leslie Ball to Norman Taylor, "RE: CDC Q and A's," July 6, 1999, https://childrenshealthdefense.org/wp-content/uploads/foia-leslie-ball-fda-no-safe-level-of-mercury.pdf.

18 "The United States Code of Federal Regulations (the CFR) requires, in general, the addition of a preservative to multi-dose vials of vaccines . . . ." See: Food and Drug Administration, "Thimerosal and Vaccines," *FDA.gov*, dated February 1, 2018, accessed March 20, 2021, https://www.fda.gov/vaccines-blood-biologics/safety-availability-biologics/thimerosal-and-vaccines. See also Code of Federal Regulations

Title 21, Chapter I, Subchapter F, Section 610.15, https://www.accessdata.fda.gov /scripts/cdrh/cfdocs/cfcfr/CFRSearch.cfm?fr=610.15.

[19] Centers for Disease Control and Prevention, "Thimerosal and Vaccines," *CDC.gov*, last reviewed August 25, 2020, accessed January 28, 2021, https://www.cdc.gov /vaccinesafety/concerns/thimerosal/index.html. Archived at https://web.archive.org /web/20210128193046/https://www.cdc.gov/vaccinesafety/concerns/thimerosal /index.html.

[20] Centers for Disease Control and Prevention, "Understanding Thimerosal, Mercury, and Vaccine Safety," *CDC.gov*, dated February 2013, accessed May 7, 2019, https:// www.cdc.gov/vaccines/hcp/patient-ed/conversations/downloads/vacsafe -thimerosal-color-office.pdf; Institute of Medicine, Immunization Safety Review Committee, *Immunization Safety Review: Vaccines and Autism* (Washington, DC: National Academies Press, 2004), pp. 135, 136, 138, https://www.nap.edu/catalog /10997/immunization-safety-review-vaccines-and-autism. The IOM was reformed in 2015 as the National Academy of Medicine.

[21] Centers for Disease Control and Prevention, "Frequently Asked Questions about Thimerosal," *CDC.gov*, updated August 28, 2015 and accessed December 20, 2018, https://www.cdc.gov/vaccinesafety/concerns/thimerosal/faqs.html; Centers for Disease Control and Prevention, "Thimerosal Publications and References," *CDC.gov*, updated October 27, 2015, and accessed December 21, 2018, https://www.cdc.gov /vaccinesafety/concerns/thimerosal/publications.html.

[22] Ball, and Pratt, "An Assessment of Thimerosal Use in Childhood Vaccines."

[23] Thomas M. Burbacher et al., "Comparison of Blood and Brain Mercury Levels in Infant Monkeys Exposed to Methylmercury or Vaccines Containing Thimerosal," *Environmental Health Perspectives*, April 21, 2005, https://www.ncbi .nlm.nih.gov/pmc/articles/PMC1280342/.

[24] José G. Dórea, "Integrating Experimental (In Vitro and In Vivo) Neurotoxicity Studies of Low-dose Thimerosal Relevant to Vaccines," *Neurochemical Research*, February 25, 2011, https://doi.org/10.1007/s11064-011-0427-0.

[25] Ibid.

The Endemic Corruption within the Medical Establishment

[1] US Food and Drug Administration, photo of FDA Building 21, Flickr, taken on November 24, 2010, accessed May 1, 2021, https://www.flickr.com/photos /fdaphotos/5204602349; United States government work, https://www.usa.gov /government-works.

[2] Anna Merlan, "Robert F. Kennedy Jr.'s Group Is a Top Buyer of Anti-Vax Facebook Ads," *Vice*, November 15, 2019, https://www.vice.com/en_us/article/43k93w/robert -f-kennedy-jrs-group-is-a-top-buyer-of-anti-vax-facebook-ads; Beth Mole, "Robert F. Kennedy Jr. is the single leading source of anti-vax ads on Facebook," *Ars Technica*, November 14, 2019, https://arstechnica.com/science/2019/11/robert-f-kennedy -jr-is-the-single-leading-source-of-anti-vax-ads-on-facebook/. For further discussion, see the following article and accompanying e-book: Jeremy R. Hammond, "CHD Responds to Accusation of Spreading 'Misinformation' on Facebook," *Children's Health Defense*, June 30, 2020, https://childrenshealthdefense.org/news/chd-responds-to -accusation-of-spreading-misinformation-on-facebook/.

3   John P.A. Ioannidis, "Why Most Published Research Findings Are False," *PLoS Medicine*, August 30, 2005, https://www.ncbi.nlm.nih.gov/pmc/articles/PMC1182327/.

4   Richard Horton, "The Dawn of McScience," *New York Review of Books*, March 11, 2004, https://www.nybooks.com/articles/2004/03/11/the-dawn-of-mcscience/.

5   Marcia Angell, "Drug Companies & Doctors: A Story of Corruption," *New York Review of Books*, January 15, 2009, https://www.nybooks.com/articles/2009/01/15/drug-companies-doctorsa-story-of-corruption/.

6   Richard Horton, "Offline: What is medicine's 5 sigma?" *The Lancet*, April 11, 2015, https://doi.org/10.1016/S0140-6736(15)60696-1.

7   Emmanuel Stamatakis, Richard Weiler, and John P.A. Ioannidis, "Undue industry influences that distort healthcare research, strategy, expenditure and practice: a review," *European Journal of Clinical Investigation*, March 25, 2013, https://doi.org/10.1111/eci.12074.

8   Michelle M. Mello, Sara Abiola, and James Colgrove, "Pharmaceutical Companies' Role in State Vaccination Policymaking: The Case of Human Papillomavirus Vaccination," *American Journal of Public Health*, April 11, 2012, https://www.ncbi.nlm.nih.gov/pmc/articles/PMC3483914/.

9   Tom Jefferson et al., "Vaccines for preventing influenza in healthy adults," *Cochrane Database of Systematic Reviews*, July 7, 2010, https://www.cochranelibrary.com/cdsr/doi/10.1002/14651858.CD001269.pub4/full. For further discussion and documentation, see: Jeremy R. Hammond, "Should You Get the Flu Shot Every Year? Don't Ask the New York Times." *JeremyRHammond.com*, February 7, 2018, https://www.jeremyrhammond.com/2018/02/07/should-you-get-the-flu-shot-every-year-dont-ask-the-new-york-times/.

10 Jeanne Lenzer, "Centers for Disease Control and Prevention: protecting the private good?" *The BMJ*, May 15, 2015, https://doi.org/10.1136/bmj.h2362.

11 CDC Foundation, "Our Story," *CDCFoundation.org*, accessed January 28, 2021, https://www.cdcfoundation.org/our-story; archived at https://web.archive.org/web/20210128234725/https://www.cdcfoundation.org/our-story.

12 CDC Foundation, "Our Partners: Corporations," *CDCFoundation.org*, accessed January 28, 2021, https://www.cdcfoundation.org/partner-list/corporations; archived at https://web.archive.org/web/20210128235535/https://www.cdcfoundation.org/partner-list/corporations.

13 Majority Staff Report of the Committee on Government Reform, "Conflicts of Interest in Vaccine Policy Making," US House of Representatives, June 15, 2000; archived at https://childrenshealthdefense.org/wp-content/uploads/conflicts-of-interest-government-reform-2000.pdf; United States Patent and Trademark Office, *Certificate Extenting Patent Term Under 35 U.S.C. § 156*, Patent No. 5,626,851, Issued May 6, 1997, https://www.uspto.gov/sites/default/files/patents/resources/terms/5626851.pdf.

14 Amy Wallace, "An Epidemic of Fear: How Panicked Parents Skipping Shots Endanger Us All," *Wired*, October 19, 2009, https://www.wired.com/2009/10/ff-waronscience/; Claudia Kalb, "Dr. Paul Offit: Debunking the Vaccine-Autism Link," *Newsweek*, October 24, 2008, https://www.newsweek.com/dr-paul-offit-debunking-vaccine-autism-link-91933.

15 Paul A. Offit, "What Would Jesus Do About Measles?" *New York Times*, February 10, 2015, https://www.nytimes.com/2015/02/10/opinion/what-would-jesus-do-about-measles.html.

16 House of Representatives, "Conflicts of Interest."
17 Jason L Schwartz, "The First Rotavirus Vaccine and the Politics of Acceptable Risk," *The Milbank Quarterly*, June 2012, https://www.ncbi.nlm.nih.gov/pmc/articles /PMC3460207/.
18 Office of Technology Transfer, "NIH Technology Licensed to Merck for HPV Vaccine," National Institutes of Health, accessed January 27, 2021, https://www.ott .nih.gov/news/nih-technology-licensed-merck-hpv-vaccine.
19 Schwartz, "The First Rotavirus Vaccine."
20 Ibid.
21 House of Representatives, "Conflicts of Interest."
22 Food and Drug Administration, "Roster of the Vaccines and Related Biological Products Advisory Committee," *FDA.gov*, dated February 9, 2021, accessed March 10, 2021, https://www.fda.gov/advisory-committees/vaccines-and-related-biological -products-advisory-committee/roster-vaccines-and-related-biological-products -advisory-committee. Archived at https://web.archive.org/web/20210311050023 /https://www.fda.gov/advisory-committees/vaccines-and-related-biological-products -advisory-committee/roster-vaccines-and-related-biological-products-advisory -committee.
23 Minority Office of the Subcommittee on Federal Financial Management, Government Information and International Security, *CDC Off Center*, United States Senate, June 2007; archived at https://www.cbsnews.com/htdocs/pdf/cdc_off_center.pdf.
24 "Former CDC head lands vaccine job at Merck," *Reuters*, December 21, 2009, https:// www.reuters.com/article/us-merck-gerberding/former-cdc-head-lands-vaccine-job -at-merck-idUSTRE5BK2K520091221.
25 United States Securities and Exchange Commission, "SEC Form 4, Statement of Changes in Beneficial Ownership for Gerberding Julie L.," *SEC.gov*, May 11, 2015, accessed January 27, 2021, https://www.sec.gov/Archives/edgar/data/310158 /000122520815011802/xslF345X01/doc4.xml. Thomas Dobrow, "Merck & Co. EVP Julie L. Gerberding Sells 38,368 Shares (MRK)," *Dakota Financial News*, May 11, 2015, archived at https://web.archive.org/web/20150528003538/http: /www.dakotafinancialnews.com/merck-co-evp-julie-l-gerberding-sells-38368-shares -mrk/159207/.
26 Merck & Co., Inc., "Julie L. Gerberding, M.D., M.P.H." *Merck.com*, accessed January 27, 2021, https://www.merck.com/leadership/julie-l-gerberding-m-d-m-p-h/.
27 Office of Inspector General, "CDC's Ethics Program for Special Government Employees on Federal Advisory," US Department of Health and Human Services, December 2009, accessed January 27, 2021, https://oig.hhs.gov/oei/reports/oei-04 -07-00260.pdf.
28 Sarah Karlin-Smith and Brianna Ehley, "Trump's top health official traded tobacco stock while leading anti-smoking efforts," *Politico*, January 30, 2018, https://www.politico .com/story/2018/01/30/cdc-director-tobacco-stocks-after-appointment-316245; Adam Cancryn and Jennifer Haberkorn, "Why the CDC director had to resign," *Politico*, January 31, 2018, https://www.politico.com/story/2018/01/31/cdc-director -resigns-fitzgerald-azar-380680.
29 Cynthia Koons, "Pfizer Names Former FDA Chief Gottlieb to Board of Directors," *Bloomberg*, June 27, 2019, https://www.bloomberg.com/news/articles /2019-06-27/pfizer-names-former-fda-chief-gottlieb-to-board-of-directors.

30 Sharyl Attkisson, "How Independent Are Vaccine Defenders?" *CBS News*, July 25, 2008, https://www.cbsnews.com/news/how-independent-are-vaccine-defenders/.

31 Christina D. Bethell et al., "A National and State Profile of Leading Health Problems and Health Care Quality for US Children: Key Insurance Disparities and Across-State Variations," *Academic Pediatrics*, May 11, 2011, https://doi.org/10.1016/j.acap.2010.08.011.

32 Grace Rattue, "Autoimmune Disease Rates Increasing," *MedicalNewsToday*, June 22, 2012, https://www.medicalnewstoday.com/articles/246960.

The Absence of Studies Examining the Safety of the CDC's Schedule

1   Dr. AJ Wakefield et al., "Ileal-lymphoid-nodular hyperplasia, non-specific colitis, and pervasive developmental disorder in children," *The Lancet*, February 28, 1998, https://doi.org/10.1016/S0140-6736(97)11096-0.

2   To cite just a few more recent examples, see: Samantha M. Matta, Elisa L. Hill-Yardin, and Peter J. Crack, "The influence of neuroinflammation in Autism Spectrum Disorder," *Brain, Behavior, and Immunity*, April 25, 2019, https://doi.org/10.1016/j.bbi.2019.04.037; John F Cryan et al., "The gut microbiome in neurological disorders," *The Lancet Neurology*, February 1, 2020, https://doi.org/10.1016/S1474-4422(19)30356-4; Sabine Hazan et al., "Shotgun Metagenomic Sequencing Identifies Dysbiosis in Triplet Sibling with Gastrointestinal Symptoms and ASD," *Children*, November 25, 2020, https://doi.org/10.3390/children7120255.

3   Editors of *The Lancet*, "Retraction—Ileal-lymphoid-nodular hyperplasia, non-specific colitis, and pervasive developmental disorder in children," *The Lancet*, February 6, 2010, https://doi.org/10.1016/S0140-6736(10)60175-4.

4   High Court of Justice, *Walker-Smith v General Medical Council*, United Kingdom, March 7, 2012, https://www.bailii.org/ew/cases/EWHC/Admin/2012/503.html. Archived at https://web.archive.org/web/20210201175222/https://www.bailii.org/ew/cases/EWHC/Admin/2012/503.html.

5   News Release, "Co-Author of *Lancet* MMR-Autism Study Exonerated on All Charges of Professional Misconduct," *Elizabeth Birt Center for Autism Law & Advocacy*, March 7, 2012, https://www.ebcala.org/areas-of-law/vaccine-law/co-author-of-lancet-mmr-autism-study-exonerated-on-all-charges-of-professional-misconduct. Archived at https://web.archive.org/web/20210119165752/https://www.ebcala.org/areas-of-law/vaccine-law/co-author-of-lancet-mmr-autism-study-exonerated-on-all-charges-of-professional-misconduct. (There is no publication date on the page, but it is shown in the source code.)

6   Wakefield et al., "Ileal-lymphoid-nodular hyperplasia."

7   Institute of Medicine, *Adverse Effects of Pertussis and Rubella Vaccines: A Report of the Committee to Review the Adverse Consequences of Pertussis and Rubella Vaccine* (Washington, DC: National Academies Press, 1991), https://doi.org/10.17226/1815.

8   Centers for Disease Control and Prevention, "Autism and Vaccines," *CDC.gov*, updated January 26, 2021, accessed February 1, 2021, https://www.cdc.gov/vaccinesafety/concerns/autism.html. Archived at https://web.archive.org/web/20210131055137/https://www.cdc.gov/vaccinesafety/concerns/autism.html. The date of last update

does not appear on the page, which shows a "last reviewed" date of August 25, 2020, but the source code reveals that it was last updated, at the time of this writing, on January 26, 2021.

9   Institute of Medicine, Immunization Safety Review Committee, *Immunization Safety Review: Vaccines and Autism* (Washington, DC: National Academies Press, 2004), pp. 135, 136, 138, https://doi.org/10.17226/10997. The IOM was reformed in 2015 as the National Academy of Medicine.

10 Institute of Medicine, Committee to Review Adverse Effects of Vaccines, *Adverse Effects of Vaccines: Evidence and Causality* (Washington, DC: National Academies Press, 2011), pp. 145–148, https://doi.org/10.17226/13164.

11 Anjali Jain et al., "Autism Occurrence by MMR Vaccine Status Among US Children With Older Siblings With and Without Autism," *JAMA*, April 21, 2015, https://doi.org/10.1001/jama.2015.3077.

12 The best example is a large study in Denmark that cited the study by Jain et al. and acknowledged the healthy user bias found in that earlier study, yet failed to account for it in their own study. See: Anders Hviid et al., "Measles, Mumps, Rubella Vaccination and Autism: A Nationwide Cohort Study," *Annals of Internal Medicine*, March 5, 2019, https://doi.org/10.7326/M18-2101.

13 Robert J. Mitkus et al., "Updated aluminum pharmacokinetics following infant exposures through diet and vaccination," *Vaccine*, November 28, 2011, https://doi.org/10.1016/j.vaccine.2011.09.124.

14 Mitkus et al., Centers for Disease Control and Prevention, "Adjuvants and Vaccines," *CDC.gov*, last reviewed August 14, 2020, accessed February 1, 2021, https://www.cdc.gov/vaccinesafety/concerns/adjuvants.html. Archived at https://web.archive.org/web/20210131131657/https://www.cdc.gov/vaccinesafety/concerns/adjuvants.html.

15 For a critical analysis of this study, see: Jean-Daniel Masson et al., "Critical analysis of reference studies on the toxicokinetics of aluminum-based adjuvants," *Journal of Inorganic Biochemistry*, December 28, 2017, https://doi.org/10.1016/j.jinorgbio.2017.12.015. See also: James Lyons-Weiler and Robert Ricketson, "Reconsideration of the immunotherapeutic pediatric safe dose levels of aluminum," *Journal of Trace Elements in Medicine and Biology*, March 8, 2018, https://doi.org/10.1016/j.jtemb.2018.02.025. On the absorption of ingested aluminum, see: Madhusudan G. Soni et al., "Safety Evaluation of Dietary Aluminum," *Regulatory Toxicology and Pharmacology*, May 25, 2002, https://doi.org/10.1006/rtph.2000.1441.

16 Department of Health and Human Services, Food and Drug Administration, "Aluminum in Large and Small Volume Parenterals Used in Total Parenteral Nutrition," Federal Register, Volume 65, Number 17, January 26, 2000, https://www.federalregister.gov/documents/2001/01/26/01-2125/aluminum-in-large-and-small-volume-parenterals-used-in-total-parenteral-nutrition-delay-of-effective.

17 For a selection of relevant studies, see: Masson et al., "Critical analysis of reference studies"; Diana L. Vargas et al., "Neuroglial Activation and Neuroinflammation in the Brain of Patients with Autism," *Annals of Neurology*, November 15, 2004, https://onlinelibrary.wiley.com/doi/abs/10.1002/ana.20315; Guillemette Crépeaux et al., "Non-linear dose-response of aluminium hydroxide adjuvant particles: Selective low dose neurotoxicity," *Toxicology*, November 28, 2016, https://doi.org/10.1016/j

.tox.2016.11.018; Marc D. Rudolph et al., "Maternal IL-6 during pregnancy can be estimated from newborn brain connectivity and predicts future working memory in offspring," *Nature Neuroscience*, April 9, 2018, https://www.nature .com/articles/s41593-018-0128-y; Dario Siniscalco et al., "Inflammation and Neuro-Immune Dysregulations in Autism Spectrum Disorders," *Pharmaceuticals*, June 4, 2018, https://www.mdpi.com/1424-8247/11/2/56/htm; Christopher Exley, "An aluminum adjuvant in a vaccine is an acute exposure to aluminum," *Journal of Trace Elements in Medicine and Biology*, September 18, 2019, https:// doi.org/10.1016/j.jtemb.2019.09.010; and Emma Shardlow, Matthew Mold, and Christopher Exley, "The interaction of aluminium-based adjuvants with THP-1 macrophages in vitro: Implications for cellular survival and systemic translocation," *Journal of Inorganic Biochemistry*, November 12, 2019, https://doi.org/10.1016/j .jinorgbio.2019.110915.

18 Lena H. Sun, "Why it's a bad idea to space out your child's vaccination shots," *Washington Post*, April 17, 2017, https://www.washingtonpost.com/news/to-your-health /wp/2017/04/17/why-its-a-bad-idea-to-space-out-your-childs-vaccination-shots/.

19 Institute of Medicine, *The Childhood Immunization Schedule and Safety* (Washington, DC: National Academies Press, 2013), p. 6, https://doi.org/10.17226/13563.

20 Jeremy R. Hammond, "WaPo Writer Brazenly Lies About Vaccine Safety, Refuses to Issue Correction," *JeremyRHammond.com*, January 23, 2018, https://www .jeremyrhammond.com/2018/01/23/wapo-writer-brazenly-lies-about-vaccine-safety -refuses-to-issue-correction/.

21 Patti Neighmond, "Schedule of Childhood Vaccines Declared Safe," *All Things Considered*, NPR, January 16, 2013, https://www.npr.org/sections/health-shots /2013/01/18/169516511/schedule-of-childhood-vaccines-declared-safe/.

22 Institute of Medicine, *The Childhood Immunization Schedule and Safety.*

23 James M. Glanz et al., "White Paper on the Study of the Safety of the Childhood Immunization Schedule for the Vaccine Safety Datalink," Centers for Disease Control and Prevention, April 17, 2016, https://stacks.cdc.gov/view/cdc/57885. The white paper was also published earlier: James M. Glanz et al., "White Paper on studying the safety of the childhood immunization schedule in the Vaccine Safety Datalink," *Vaccine*, January 29, 2016, https://doi.org/10.1016/j.vaccine.2015.10.082. I did not determine whether the versions are identical or significant revisions were made in the April publication reviewed here.

Dr. Paul's Awakening

1 Paul Thomas, MD, "A CRAZY DAY IN THE LIFE of a Busy Pediatrician (EXTENDED CUT)," YouTube, March 2, 2021, accessed May 1, 2021, https:// www.youtube.com/watch?v=MgYotcWMQeM. Screenshot from the video.

2 The website of the Autism Research Institute is https://www.autism.org/. The website of the Medical Academy of Pediatric Special Needs is https://www.medmaps.org/.

3 Yehuda Shoenfeld, Nancy Agmon-Levin, Lucija Tomljenovic, *Vaccines and Autoimmunity* (Hoboken, NJ: Wiley-Blackwell, May 2015), https://www.wiley.com/en-us /Vaccines+and+Autoimmunity-p-9781118663493; Sheba International, "Professor Yehuda Shoenfeld, MD, FRCP," *ShebaOnline.org*, accessed February 1, 2021, https://

www.shebaonline.org/doctors/yehuda-shoenfeld/. Archived at https://web.archive.org/web/20210202033807/https://www.shebaonline.org/doctors/yehuda-shoenfeld/. The search result for Shoenfeld's author ID on PubMed was accessed on February 1, 2021, https://pubmed.ncbi.nlm.nih.gov/?term=Shoenfeld%20Y&cauthor_id=26275795. Archived at https://web.archive.org/web/20210202034207if_/https://pubmed.ncbi.nlm.nih.gov/?term=Shoenfeld+Y&cauthor_id=26275795.

Oregon State's Rejection of the Right to Informed Consent

1 Oregon Health Authority, "Nonmedical Vaccine Exemptions," Vaccine Education Module, Oregon.gov, module accessed January 12, 2021, https://www.oregon.gov/OHA/PH/PreventionWellness/VaccinesImmunization/GettingImmunized/Pages/nonmedical-exemption.aspx. Archived at https://web.archive.org/web/20210107103455/https://www.oregon.gov/OHA/PH/PreventionWellness/VaccinesImmunization/GettingImmunized/Pages/nonmedical-exemption.aspx. Screenshot from the introduction video of the Vaccine Education Module.

2 ORS 677.097—Procedure to obtain informed consent of patient, https://www.oregonlaws.org/ors/677.097.

3 ORS 433.267—Immunization of school children, https://www.oregonlaws.org/ors/433.267; Oregon Health Authority, "Oregon School Immunization Law Summary, 2020," Oregon.gov, April 30, 2018, accessed February 2, 2021, https://www.oregon.gov/oha/PH/PREVENTIONWELLNESS/VACCINESIMMUNIZATION/GETTINGIMMUNIZED/Documents/SchLawSum.pdf. Archived at https://web.archive.org/web/20210202175722/https://www.oregon.gov/oha/PH/PREVENTIONWELLNESS/VACCINESIMMUNIZATION/GETTINGIMMUNIZED/Documents/SchLawSum.pdf.

4 Oregon Health Authority, "Oregon School Immunization Law Summary, 2020."

5 Dr. Andrew Walter Zimmerman, Affidavit, September 7, 2018. Published by Sharyl Attkisson, "Dr. Andrew Zimmerman's full Affidavit on alleged link between vaccines and autism that U.S. govt. covered up," *SharylAttkisson.com*, January 6, 2019, https://sharylattkisson.com/2019/01/06/dr-andrew-zimmermans-full-affidavit-on-alleged-link-between-vaccines-and-autism-that-u-s-govt-covered-up/, archived at https://web.archive.org/web/20210202210041/https://sharylattkisson.com/2019/01/dr-andrew-zimmermans-full-affidavit-on-alleged-link-between-vaccines-and-autism-that-u-s-govt-covered-up/.

6 Attkisson, "Dr. Andrew Zimmerman's full Affidavit." See also: Sharyl Attkisson, "The Vaccination Debate," *Full Measure*, January 6, 2019, https://fullmeasure.news/news/cover-story/the-vaccination-debate. Archived at https://web.archive.org/web/20210119151531/http://fullmeasure.news/news/cover-story/the-vaccination-debate; Sharyl Attkisson, "How a pro-vaccine doctor reopened debate about link to autism," *The Hill*, January 13, 2019, https://thehill.com/opinion/healthcare/425061-how-a-pro-vaccine-doctor-reopened-debate-about-link-to-autism. Archived at https://web.archive.org/web/20210202210354/https://thehill.com/opinion/healthcare/425061-how-a-pro-vaccine-doctor-reopened-debate-about-link-to-autism; Children's Health Defense, "Robert F. Kennedy, Jr. Demands the Office of the Inspector General and Congress Investigate Department of Justice for Fraud and Obstruction

of Justice," *PRNewswire*, January 14, 2019, https://www.prnewswire.com/news
-releases/robert-f-kennedy-jr-demands-the-office-of-the-inspector-general-and
-congress-investigate-department-of-justice-for-fraud-and-obstruction-of
-justice-300777802.html. Archived at https://web.archive.org/web/20200410195746
/https://www.prnewswire.com/news-releases/robert-f-kennedy-jr-demands-the-office
-of-the-inspector-general-and-congress-investigate-department-of-justice-for-fraud
-and-obstruction-of-justice-300777802.html.

[7] David Kirby, "The Vaccine-Autism Court Document Every American Should
Read," *Huffington Post*, February 26, 2008, https://www.huffpost.com/entry/the
-vaccineautism-court-d_n_88558. Note that the rebranded *HuffPo* has now censored
this article from their website on the grounds that vaccines are "safe and effective", and any
content that suggests anything differently cannot be tolerated. I have archived a copy here:
https://www.jeremyrhammond.com/wp-content/uploads/2019/10/080226-Vaccine
-Autism-Court-Document-Kirby-HuffPost.pdf.

[8] *House Call With Dr. Sanjay Gupta*, CNN, March 29, 2008, https://transcripts.cnn
.com/TRANSCRIPTS/0803/29/hcsg.01.html. Archived at https://web.archive
.org/web/20080517120027/https://transcripts.cnn.com/TRANSCRIPTS/0803/29
/hcsg.01.html.

[9] Sharyl Attkisson, "CDC: 'Possibility' that vaccines rarely trigger autism," December 10,
2018, *SharylAttkisson.com*, https://sharylattkisson.com/2018/12/10/cdc-possibility
-that-vaccines-rarely-trigger-autism/. Archived at https://web.archive.org/web/201812
12120426/https://sharylattkisson.com/2018/12/10/cdc-possibility-that-vaccines
-rarely-trigger-autism/.

[10] Oregon Health Authority, Vaccine Education Module.

[11] James D. Cherry, "The 112-Year Odyssey of Pertussis and Pertussis Vaccines—
Mistakes Made and Implications for the Future," *Journal of the Pediatric Infectious
Diseases Society*, February 22, 2019, https://doi.org/10.1093/jpids/piz005.

[12] Jason M. Warfel, Lindsey I. Zimmerman, and Tod J. Merkel, "Acellular pertussis
vaccines protect against disease but fail to prevent infection and transmission in a
nonhuman primate model," *PNAS*, January 14, 2014, https://doi.org/10.1073
/pnas.1314688110; Food and Drug Administration, "FDA study helps provide an
understanding of rising rates of whooping cough and response to vaccination," *FDA
.gov*, November 27, 2013, archived at https://web.archive.org/web/20131129223213
/https://www.fda.gov/NewsEvents/Newsroom/PressAnnouncements/ucm376937
.htm; Sabrina Tavernise, "Whooping Cough Study May Offer Clue on Surge,"
New York Times, November 25, 2013, https://www.nytimes.com/2013/11/26/health
/study-finds-vaccinated-baboons-can-still-carry-whooping-cough.html.

[13] Institute of Medicine, *The Childhood Immunization Schedule and Safety*. Again, "studies
designed to examine the long-term effects of the cumulative number of vaccines or
other aspects of the immunization schedule have not been conducted."

Punishing Doctors for Serving Their Patients Rather Than the State

[1] Dr. Richard Pan, photo of Dr. Richard Pan with a child, Flickr, taken on April 6,
2014, accessed May 1, 2021, https://www.flickr.com/photos/49307181@N06

/14001841794. Licensed under Creative Commons Attribution-ShareAlike 2.0 Generic (CC BY-SA 2.0), https://creativecommons.org/licenses/by-sa/2.0/.

2   Paul L. Delamater et al., "Elimination of Nonmedical Immunization Exemptions in California and School-Entry Vaccine Status," *Pediatrics*, May 31, 2019, https://doi .org/10.1542/peds.2018-3301.

3   Lewis First, "Eliminating Nonmedical Immunization Exemptions in California: Is It Working?" *Journals Blog* (American Academy of Pediatrics), May 22, 2019, https://www.aappublications.org/news/2019/05/22/eliminating-nonmedical -immunization-exemptions-in-california-is-it-working-pediatrics-5-22-19.   Archived at   https://web.archive.org/web/20200317222758/https://www.aappublications.org /news/2019/05/22/eliminating-nonmedical-immunization-exemptions-in-california -is-it-working-pediatrics-5-22-19.

4   Office of California State Senator Dr. Richard Pan, "Dr. Richard Pan Introduces SB 276 to Combat Fake Medical Exemptions that Put Children and Communities at Risk," Press Release, California State Senate, March 26, 2019, https://sd06 .senate.ca.gov/news/2019-03-26-dr-richard-pan-introduces-sb-276-combat -fake-medical-exemptions-put-children-and.   Archived   at   https://web.archive.org /web/20190425062031/https://sd06.senate.ca.gov/news/2019-03-26-dr-richard -pan-introduces-sb-276-combat-fake-medical-exemptions-put-children-and.

5   California State Senate, *Senate Bill No. 276*, approved by the governor September 9,   2019,   https://leginfo.legislature.ca.gov/faces/billTextClient.xhtml?bill_id=2019 -20200SB276; Katherine Drabiak, "California law to restrict medical vaccine exemptions raises thorny questions over control," *The Conversation*, September 24, 2019, https://theconversation.com/california-law-to-restrict-medical-vaccine-exemptions -raises-thorny-questions-over-control-123563.

6   Richard J. Pan and Dorit Rubinstein Reiss, "Vaccine Medical Exemptions Are a Delegated Public Health Authority," *Pediatrics*, November 2018, https://doi .org/10.1542/peds.2018-2009.

7   Jim Miller, "Drug companies donated millions to California lawmakers before vaccine debate," *The Sacramento Bee*, June 18, 2015, https://www.sacbee.com/news/politics -government/capitol-alert/article24913978.html.

8   Robert W. Sears, *The Vaccine Book: Making the Right Decision for Your Child* (New York: Little, Brown and Company, 2007).

9   Paul A. Offit and Charlotte A. Moser, "The Problem With Dr Bob's Alternative Vaccine Schedule," *Pediatrics*, December 29, 2008, https://doi.org/10.1542/peds.2008-2189.

10   Medical Board of California, "In the Matter of the Accusation Against: Robert William Sears, M.D.," *MBC.CA.gov*, June 27, 2018, archived at https://web.archive.org /web/20181103140437/http://www2.mbc.ca.gov/BreezePDL/document.aspx ?path=%5CDIDOCS%5C20180627%5CDMRAAAGL14%5C&did =AAAGL180627201150927.DID.

11   Rong-Gong Lin II, Soumya Karlamangla, and Rosanna Xia, "California wants to pull this doctor's license. Here's how it's sparked a new battle over child vaccinations," *Los Angeles Times*, September 12, 2016, http://www.latimes.com/local/lanow/la-me-sears -vaccine-20160909-snap-story.html.

12   Soumya Karlamangla, "Leading vaccine skeptic Dr. Bob Sears placed on probation after exempting 2-year-old boy from all childhood vaccinations," *Los Angeles Times*, June 29,

2018,   http://www.latimes.com/local/california/la-me-ln-sears-license-20180629
-story.html. See also Medical Board of California, "In the Matter of the Accusation."

13 Salini Mohanty et al., "Experience With Medical Exemptions After a Change in
Vaccine Exemption Policy in California," *Pediatrics*, November 1, 2018, https://doi
.org/10.1542/peds.2018-1051.

Dr. Paul's Vaccine-Friendly Plan

1 Robert A. Bednarczyk, Dzifa Adjaye-Gbewonyo, and Saad B. Omer, "Safety of
influenza immunization during pregnancy for the fetus and the neonate," *American
Journal of Obstetrics & Gynecology*, September 2012, https://doi.org/10.1016/j
.ajog.2012.07.002.

2 I'm quoting here specifically from the insert for GlaxoSmithKline's Fluarix
product, but this warning is standard in this or similar wording in all inactived
influenza vaccine package inserts. GlaxoSmithKline Biologicals, FLUARIX
(Influenza Vaccine) Package Insert, FDA.gov, accessed December 5, 2018, https://
www.fda.gov/downloads/BiologicsBloodVaccines/Vaccines/ApprovedProducts
/UCM335392.pdf. For the parent page linking to this document, see: https://www
.fda.gov/BiologicsBloodVaccines/Vaccines/ApprovedProducts/ucm112850.htm.   For
further discussion and documentation related to influenza vaccination of pregnant
women, see: Jeremy R. Hammond, "The CDC's Criminal Recommendation for a
Flu Shot During Pregnancy," *JeremyRHammond.com*, May 14, 2019, https://www
.jeremyrhammond.com/2019/05/14/the-cdcs-criminal-recommendation-for-a-flu
-shot-during-pregnancy/.

The Oregon Medical Board Takes Aim at Dr. Paul

1 Photo of a medical professional with a pregnant woman, Max Pixel, accessed May
1, 2021, https://www.maxpixel.net/Assessment-Consultation-Pregnancy-Medicine
-Pregnant-3486590. Licensed under Creative Commons CC0 Public Domain,
https://creativecommons.org/share-your-work/public-domain/cc0.

2 Oregon Medical Board, letter of complaint to Dr. Paul Thomas, December 26,
2018.

3 Letter from Larry A. Brisbee to Oregon Medical Board Investigator Mr. Jason
Bommels, January 11, 2019.

4 GlaxoSmithKline Biologicals, "Fluarix Influenza Virus Vaccine," Package Insert,
FDA.gov, accessed February 27, 2021, https://www.fda.gov/media/84804/
download. See also the parent page: https://www.fda.gov/vaccines-blood-biologics/
vaccines/fluarix. The full list of vaccines licensed for use in the US with links to
inserts is at https://www.fda.gov/vaccines-blood-biologics/vaccines/vaccines-
licensed-use-united-states.

5 Sanofi Pasteur, Inc, "Fluzone Influenza Virus Vaccine," Package Insert, *FDA.gov*,
accessed February 27, 2021, https://www.fda.gov/media/116102/download. See
also the parent page: https://www.fda.gov/vaccines-blood-biologics/vaccines/fluzone
-fluzone-high-dose-and-fluzone-intradermal.

6   Seqirus Vaccines Limited, "Fluvirin Influenza Virus Vaccine," Package Insert, *FDA
    .gov*, accessed February 27, 2021, https://www.fda.gov/media/75156/download. See
    also the parent page: https://www.fda.gov/vaccines-blood-biologics/vaccines/fluvirin.

7   Kana Ozaki et al., "Maternal immune activation induces sustained changes in fetal
    microglia motility," *Nature*, December 7, 2020, https://doi.org/10.1038/s41598-020
    -78294-2.

8   Burbacher et al., "Comparison of Blood and Brain Mercury Levels."

9   Sanofi Pasteur, Ltd, "Tetanus Toxoid, Reduced Diphtheria Toxoid and Acellular
    Pertussis Vaccine, Adsorbed," Package Insert, *FDA.gov*, accessed February 27, 2021,
    https://www.fda.gov/media/119862/download. See also the parent page: https://
    www.fda.gov/vaccines-blood-biologics/vaccines/adacel.

10 GlaxoSmithKline Biologicals, "Tetanus Toxoid, Reduced Diphtheria Toxoid and
    Acellular Pertussis Vaccine, Adsorbed," Package Insert, *FDA.gov*, accessed February
    27, 2021, https://www.fda.gov/media/124002/download. See also the parent page:
    https://www.fda.gov/vaccines-blood-biologics/vaccines/boostrix.

11 Oregon Medical Board, letter to Dr. Paul Thomas, December 26, 2018.

12 Institute of Medicine, *The Childhood Immunization Schedule and Safety*. Again, "studies
    designed to examine the long-term effects of the cumulative number of vaccines or
    other aspects of the immunization schedule have not been conducted."

13 James Lyons-Weiler and Paul Thomas, "Correction: Lyons-Weiler, J., et al. Relative
    Incidence of Office Visits and Cumulative Rates of Billed Diagnoses along the Axis
    of Vaccination. *Int. J. Environ. Res. Public Health* 2020, *17*, 8674," January 22, 2012,
    https://doi.org/10.3390/ijerph18030936.

14 Ibid.

15 Anecdotally, when Thomas said this, it reminded me of an experience with a
    hairdresser who, as she was cutting my hair, told me how she had taken her son in to
    see the doctor because she was so concerned about his behavior, such as going around
    pounding his head into the walls. "But he said, 'That's *normal.*'" In the way that
    she said it, she was communicating that this went against her own gut instinct that
    something was wrong. There was a sense of frustration about the fact that that was the
    doctor's reaction when told that her child *was going around banging his head into the
    wall.* I sympathized by agreeing that this was *not* normal behavior but stopped short
    of sharing my opinion about what might possibly be the cause.

A Local Newspaper Joins in the Attacks on Dr. Paul

1   Rachel Monahan, "Pediatrician Paul Thomas Has 15,000 Patients—and He Tells Them
    the Measles Vaccine Might Cause Autism," *Willamette Week*, March 20, 2019, https://
    www.wweek.com/news/2019/03/20/pediatrician-paul-thomas-has-15000-patients
    -and-he-tells-them-the-measles-vaccine-might-cause-autism/. Archived at https://
    web.archive.org/web/20210208184154/https://www.wweek.com/news/2019/03/20
    /pediatrician-paul-thomas-has-15000-patients-and-he-tells-them-the-measles
    -vaccine-might-cause-autism/.

2   Ibid.

3   Ibid.

4   Ibid.

5   Ibid.

6   WW Staff, "Support Local Journalism," *Willamette Week,* accessed February
    8, 2021, https://www.wweek.com/fund/. Archived at https://web.archive.org
    /web/20210208221917/https://www.wweek.com/fund/.

7   Pediatric Associates of the Northwest, "Jay S. Rosenbloom MD, PhD, FAAP,"
    PortlandPediatric.com, accessed February 8, 2021, http://www.portlandpediatric
    .com/physicians-and-providers/jay-srosenbloom. Archived at https://web.archive.org
    /web/20200928122408/http://www.portlandpediatric.com/physicians-and
    -providers/jay-srosenbloom; Children's Health Foundation, "Jay Rosenbloom, MD,
    PhD," *CH-Foundation.org,* accessed February 8, 2021, https://ch-foundation.org
    /about/jay-rosenbloom/. Archived at https://web.archive.org/web/20210208183052
    /https://ch-foundation.org/about/jay-rosenbloom/.

8   CDC, "Thimerosal and Vaccines," Institute of Medicine, *Immunization Safety Review.*
    Burbacher et al., "Comparison of Blood and Brain Mercury Levels."

While CDC Stalls, Independent Researchers Forge Ahead

1   Amanda Mills, USCDCP, photo of a baby appearing to receive an injection,
    Pixnio, accessed May 1, 2021, https://pixnio.com/science/medical-science
    /baby-was-receiving-his-scheduled-vaccine-injection-in-his-right-thigh-muscle
    -ie-intramuscular-injection. Licensed under CC0 for Public Domain Dedication,
    https://creativecommons.org/licenses/publicdomain/.

2   Anthony R Mawson et al., "Pilot comparative study on the health of vaccinated
    and unvaccinated 6- to 12-year old U.S. children," *Journal of Translational Science,*
    April 24, 2017, https://doi.org/10.15761/JTS.1000186.

3   IPAK's website is http://ipaknowledge.org/. Dr. James Lyons-Weiler's blog is https://
    jameslyonsweiler.com/. The book is James Lyons-Weiler, *The Environmental and
    Genetic Causes of Autism* (New York, NY: Skyhorse Publishing, November 2016),
    https://www.skyhorsepublishing.com/9781510710863/the-environmental-and
    -genetic-causes-of-autism/.

4   Grant McFarland et al., "Acute exposure and chronic retention of aluminum in three
    vaccine schedules and effects of genetic and environmental variation," *Journal of Trace
    Elements in Medicine in Biology,* December 5, 2019 (in print March 2020), https://
    doi.org/10.1016/j.jtemb.2019.126444.

5   Ibid.

6   Ibid.

7   Ibid.

8   Ibid.

9   Brian S. Hooker and Neil Z. Miller, "Analysis of health outcomes in vaccinated
    and unvaccinated children: Developmental delays, asthma, ear infections and
    gastrointestinal disorders," *SAGE Open Medicine,* May 27, 2020, https://doi.org/10.1
    -177%2F2050312120925344.

10 Ibid.

Measuring the Wrong Health Outcomes

1   Paul Thomas, MD, "A CRAZY DAY IN THE LIFE." Screenshot from the video.
2   Centers for Disease Control and Prevention, "Vaccines for Children Program (VFC)," *CDC.gov*, last reviewed February 18, 2016, accessed February 11, 2021, https://www.cdc.gov/vaccines/programs/vfc/index.html.
3   Rachel Monahan, "Vaccine-Doubting Oregon Doctor Loses Medicaid Funding," *Willamette Week*, August 7, 2019, https://www.wweek.com/news/2019/08/07/vaccine-doubting-oregon-doctor-loses-medicaid-funding/. Archived at https://web.archive.org/web/20210211192646/https://www.wweek.com/news/2019/08/07/vaccine-doubting-oregon-doctor-loses-medicaid-funding/.
4   Dr. Paul Thomas, letter to Oregon Medical Board Investigator Mr. Jason Boemmels, August 27, 2019.
5   Letter to Dr. Paul Thomas from a major private provider, September 15, 2020.
6   Centers for Disease Control and Prevention, "Hepatitis B Virus: A Comprehensive Strategy for Eliminating Transmission in the United States Through Universal Childhood Vaccination: Recommendations of the Immunization Practices Advisory Committee (ACIP)," *MMWR*, November 22, 1991, https://www.cdc.gov/mmwr/preview/MMWRhtml/00033405.htm. For further discussion and documentation, see: Jeremy R. Hammond, "Why Does the CDC Recommend Hepatitis B Vaccination for Infants?" *Children's Health Defense*, April 2, 2019, https://childrenshealthdefense.org/child-health-topics/why-does-the-cdc-recommend-hepatitis-b-vaccination-for-infants/.
7   James Lyons-Weiler, "IPAK Vaxxed vs. Unvaxxed Study," *IPAK*, updated December 6, 2020, accessed February 11, 2020, http://ipaknowledge.org/. Archived at https://web.archive.org/web/20210211210314/http://ipaknowledge.org/.
8   Jonathan Duffy, "Advisory Commission on Childhood Vaccines (ACCV) meeting," Immunization Safety Office, Centers for Disease Control and Prevention, *HRSA.gov*, December 3, 2020, https://www.hrsa.gov/sites/default/files/hrsa/advisory-committees/vaccines/meetings/2020/cdc-safety-child-immunization-schedule.pdf.

How the Media Reported Dr. Paul's Suspension

1   Giggel, photo of 200 Liberty Street, Wikimedia Commons, taken on October 30, 2015, accessed May 1, 2021, https://commons.wikimedia.org/wiki/File:NYC_-_200_Liberty_Street_-_Winter_Garden_-_200_Vesey_Street_-_Goldman_Sachs_World_Headquarters_-_panoramio.jpg. Licensed under Creative Commons Attribution 3.0 Unported (CC BY 3.0), https://creativecommons.org/licenses/by/3.0/deed.en.
2   Rachel Monahan, "Prominent Anti-Vaccine Pediatrician Dr. Paul Thomas Has License Suspended by the Oregon Medical Board," *Willamette Week*, December 6, 2020, https://www.wweek.com/news/state/2020/12/05/prominent-anti-vaccine-pediatrician-dr-paul-thomas-has-license-suspended-by-the-oregon-medical-board/.
3   Lizzy Acker, "Anti-vaccine Portland pediatrician's license suspended; cases include boy hospitalized with tetanus," Oregon Live, December 8, 2020, https://www.oregonlive.com/portland/2020/12/anti-vaccine-portland-pediatricians-license-suspended-cases-include-boy-hospitalized-with-tetanus.html. Archived at https://web.archive.org

/web/20210110215034/https://www.oregonlive.com/portland/2020/12/anti
-vaccine-portland-pediatricians-license-suspended-cases-include-boy-hospitalized
-with-tetanus.html.

4   Lizzy Acker, "Remember the kid who was hospitalized for two months with
    tetanus . . .," *Twitter*, December 7, 2020, https://twitter.com/lizzzyacker/status
    /1336047276913901568.

5   Jeremy R. Hammond, "Are you aware that a peer-reviewed study...," *Twitter*, December
    8, 2020, https://twitter.com/jeremyrhammond/status/1336435885185921030.

6   James Lyons-Weiler, "Correct. This was retaliation for a study . . .," *Twitter*, December
    8, 2020, https://twitter.com/lifebiomedguru/status/1336454273211699202.

7   Tom Hallman Jr., "Love builds the Thomas family: from Africa to Portland, from
    five kids to nine," Oregon Live, October 25, 2009, https://www.oregonlive.com
    /portland/2009/10/love_builds_the_thomas_family.html. Archived at https://web
    .archive.org/web/20210216192000/https://www.oregonlive.com/portland/2009/10
    /love_builds_the_thomas_family.html.

8   Anonymous, "Pediatrician's license suspended in Oregon over vaccines," *Associated
    Press*, December 8, 2020, https://apnews.com/article/health-paul-thomas-portland
    -tetanus-oregon-48d917259b7985e6e335c67773507c62.

9   Oregon Medical Board, "Order of Emergency Suspension."

The Oregon Medical Board's Accusations

1   Paul Thomas, MD, "I MET WITH THE MEDICAL BOARD ABOUT MY
    SUSPENDED LICENSE…," YouTube, March 8, 2021, https://www.youtube.com
    /watch?v=Z-ZVtE0NCxs. Screenshot taken from the video.

2   Ibid.

3   ORS 677.190—Grounds for suspending, revoking or refusing to grant license,
    registration or certification, https://www.oregonlaws.org/ors/677.190. ORS 677.188
    —Definitions for ORS 677.190, https://www.oregonlaws.org/ors/677.188.

4   Ibid.; ORS 677.097.

5   Oregon Rule 333-050-0050—Immunization Requirements, https://oregon.public
    .law/rules/oar_333-050-0050.

6   Oregon Medical Board, "Order of Emergency Suspension."

7   Nicholas Bakalar, "Pertussis Passed to Newborns From Siblings," *New York Times*,
    September 7, 2015, https://well.blogs.nytimes.com/2015/09/07/pertussis-passed-to
    -newborns-from-siblings.

8   Rotem Lapidot and Christopher J. Gill, "The Pertussis resurgence: putting together
    the pieces of the puzzle," *Tropical Diseases, Travel Medicine and Vaccines*, December 12,
    2016, https://www.ncbi.nlm.nih.gov/pmc/articles/PMC5530967/.

9   Food and Drug Administration, "FDA study helps provide an understanding of rising
    rates of whooping cough and response to vaccination," *FDA.gov*, November 27, 2013,
    https://www.fda.gov/NewsEvents/Newsroom/PressAnnouncements/ucm376937
    .htm. Archived at https://web.archive.org/web/20160302154650/https://www.fda
    .gov/NewsEvents/Newsroom/PressAnnouncements/ucm376937.htm. See also: Jason
    M. Warfel, Lindsey I. Zimmerman, and Tod J. Merkel, "Acellular pertussis vaccines

protect against disease but fail to prevent infection and transmission in a nonhuman primate model," *PNAS*, January 14, 2014, https://doi.org/10.1073/pnas.1314688110.

10 Sabrina Tavernise, "Whooping Cough Study May Offer Clue on Surge," *New York Times*, November 25, 2013, https://www.nytimes.com/2013/11/26/health/study -finds-vaccinated-baboons-can-still-carry-whooping-cough.html.

11 Stacey W. Martin et al., "Pertactin-Negative *Bordetella pertussis* Strains: Evidence for a Possible Selective Advantage," *Clinical Infectious Diseases*, January 15, 2015, https://doi.org/10.1093/cid/ciu788.

12 Lapidot and Gill, "The Pertussis resurgence."

13 Ibid.

14 Centers for Disease Control and Prevention, "Meeting of the Board of Scientific Counselors, Office of Infectious Diseases," *CDC.gov*, December 11-12, 2013, https://www.cdc.gov/maso/facm/pdfs/BSCOID/2013121112_BSCOID_Minutes.pdf. Archived at https://web.archive.org/web/20150322163051/https://www.cdc.gov /maso/facm/pdfs/BSCOID/2013121112_BSCOID_Minutes.pdf. See also: Martin et al., "Pertactin-Negative *Bordetella pertussis* Strains."

15 Cherry, "The 112-Year Odyssey of Pertussis and Pertussis Vaccines."

16 Oregon Medical Board, "Order of Emergency Suspension."

17 Mayo Clinic Staff, "Fever," *Mayo Clinic*, accessed February 19, 2021, https://www .mayoclinic.org/diseases-conditions/fever/symptoms-causes/syc-20352759. Archived at https://web.archive.org/web/20210215171515/https://www.mayoclinic.org/diseases -conditions/fever/symptoms-causes/syc-20352759.

18 Mayo Clinic Staff, "Kawasaki disease," *Mayo Clinic*, accessed February 19, 2021, https://www.mayoclinic.org/diseases-conditions/kawasaki-disease/symptoms-causes /syc-20354598. Archived at https://web.archive.org/web/20210219223557/https:// www.mayoclinic.org/diseases-conditions/kawasaki-disease/symptoms-causes/syc -20354598.

19 Mayo Clinic, "Fever."

20 Judith A. Guzman-Cottrill, "Tetanus in an Unvaccinated Child—Oregon, 2017," *MMWR*, March 8, 2019, http://dx.doi.org/10.15585/mmwr.mm6809a3.

21 Oregon Medical Board, "Order of Emergency Suspension."

22 Ibid.

23 Lyons-Weiler and Thomas, "Relative Incidence of Office Visits."

24 Oregon Medical Board, "Order of Emergency Suspension."

25 Anecdotally, I have myself suffered from chronic gut problems that finally manifested in food hypersensitivities that caused a wide range of symptoms, including hives and other types of itchy rash and migraines. Doctors diagnosed me with "irritable bowel syndrome" (IBS), which is essentially their way of saying you have gut problems for which they don't understand the cause. After spending much time researching the medical literature for answers, I diagnosed myself with "leaky gut", otherwise known in the literature as intestinal hyperpermeability. When I told doctors I had leaky gut, they literally mocked me, denying this condition's existence despite its being completely uncontroversial in the literature. They refused to listen to me and instead wasted my time making me jump through their hoops. For example, they insisted I had typical "food allergies", which I denied, pointing out

that I had never had any reactions to foods for most of my life. I tested negative for IgE-mediated food allergies using both blood and skin-prick tests. Undeterred by their idiocy, I successfully treated myself in large part by doing an elimination diet to identify my trigger foods, which included *all* grains, dairy, soy, and alcohol. I also learned to avoid all foods that are GMO (genetically modified organism) or contain ingredients derived from GMO crops. As much as feasible, we switched to organic products. We minimize our intake of processed foods and aim to get most of our nutrition from whole foods, supplementing as we feel necessary. For example, I took zinc regularly for a time to help with the restoration of my gut lining, and I successfully treated the sensation of finger tingling or numbness by supplementing methylcobalamin (a more bioavailable form of vitamin B12), since I was evidently not getting enough from foods due to malabsorption. We also support a diversified gut microbiome through diet, such as eating homemade sauerkraut, kimchi, and kombucha. Since my gut has healed considerably, I no longer have chronic diarrhea, itchy rashes, or severe migraines. I have even been able to reintroduce foods that I was previously reacting to, such as rice. I can even tolerate small amounts of organic wheat now, although I continue to limit my intake, since gluten itself can contribute to leaky gut by triggering the release of zonulin, which modulates the tight junctions of the gut cell lining, which helps to explain the phenomenon of nonceliac gluten sensitivity. There is an abundance of literature on this, but see, for one example: Alessio Fasano, "All disease begins in the (leaky) gut: role of zonulin-mediated gut permeability in the pathogenesis of some chronic inflammatory diseases," *F1000Research*, January 31, 2020, https://www.ncbi.nlm.nih.gov/pmc/articles/PMC6996528/.

[26] L Perelmutter, "IgG4: non-IgE mediated atopic disease," *Annals of Allergy*, February 1984, https://pubmed.ncbi.nlm.nih.gov/6364895/.

[27] Gerard E. Mullin et al., "Testing for Food Reactions: The Good, the Bad, and the Ugly," *Nutrition in Clinical Practice*, April 22, 2010, https://doi.org/10.1177/0884533610362696.

[28] Anna Nowak-Węgrzyn et al., "Non-IgE-mediated gastrointestinal food allergy," *Journal of Allergy and Clinical Immunology*, May 1, 2015, https://doi.org/10.1016/j.jaci.2015.03.025.

[29] Francis Coucke, "Food intolerance in patients with manifest autoimmunity. Observational study," *Autoimmunity Reviews*, September 11, 2018, https://doi.org/10.1016/j.autrev.2018.05.011.

[30] Lori Connors et al., "Non-IgE-mediated food hypersensitivity," *Allergy, Asthma & Clinical Immunology*, September 12, 2018, https://www.ncbi.nlm.nih.gov/pmc/articles/PMC6157279/.

[31] James F Geiselman, "The Clinical Use of IgG Food Sensitivity Testing with Migraine Headache Patients: a Literature Review," *Current Pain and Headache Reports*, August 2019, https://doi.org/10.1007/s11916-019-0819-4.

[32] Roxane Labrosse, François Graham, and Jean-Christoph Caubet, "Non-IgE-Mediated Gastrointestinal Food Allergies in Children: An Update," *Nutrients*, July 14, 2020, https://www.ncbi.nlm.nih.gov/pmc/articles/PMC7400851/.

[33] Oregon Medical Board, "Order of Emergency Suspension."

[34] Harvey W. Kaufman and Zhen Chen, "Trends in Laboratory Rotavirus Detection: 2003 to 2014," *Pediatrics*, September 30, 2016, https://doi.org/10.1542/peds.2016 -1173.

[35] Raúl Pérez-Ortín, "Rotavirus symptomatic infection among unvaccinated and vaccinated children in Valencia, Spain," *BMC Infectious Diseases*, November 27, 2019, https://www.ncbi.nlm.nih.gov/pmc/articles/PMC6880582/.

[36] Kaufman and Chen, "Trends in Laboratory Rotavirus Detection."

[37] Eleanor Burnett, Ben A. Lopman, and Umesh D. Parashar, "Potential for a booster dose of rotavirus vaccine to further reduce diarrhea mortality," *Vaccine*, November 17, 2017, https://www.ncbi.nlm.nih.gov/pmc/articles/PMC5841463/.

[38] L.J. White et al., "Rotavirus within day care centres in Oxfordshire, UK: characterization of partial immunity," *Journal of the Royal Society Interface*, May 13, 2008, https://doi.org/10.1098/rsif.2008.0115.

[39] Burnett et al., "Potential for a booster dose of rotavirus vaccine."

[40] Andrew Clark et al., "Efficacy of live oral rotavirus vaccines by duration of follow-up: a meta-regression of randomized controlled trials," *Lancet Infectious Diseases*, June 6, 2019, https://doi.org/10.1016/S1473-3099(19)30126-4.

[41] Ibid. The reasons for the disparity in immune responses to rotavirus between wealthy and poor countries are "not well understood", the study noted, but hypotheses for lower "immunogenicity" of vaccines in developing countries include "interference by maternal antibodies, interference by oral polio vaccines, neutralizing factors present in breastmilk, malnutrition, other enteric coinfections, rotavirus strain diversity, and HIV infection. Competition in the gut has also been proposed as a reason for the lower performance of oral polio vaccine in resource-poor settings." Research was also being done "to assess the role of maternal antibodies and gut microbiota in the immune response to rotavirus vaccines" in infants.

[42] Daniel C. Payne et al., "Sibling Transmission of Vaccine-Derived Rotavirus (RotaTeq) Associated with Rotavirus Gastroenteritis," *Pediatrics*, February 1, 2010, https://doi .org/10.1542/peds.2009-1901.

[43] Luis Rivera, "Horizontal transmission of a human rotavirus vaccine strain—A randomized, placebo-controlled study in twins," *Vaccine*, October 18, 2011, https:// doi.org/10.1016/j.vaccine.2011.10.015.

[44] Sylvie Escolano, Catherine Hill, and Pascale Tubert-Bitter, "Intussusception risk after RotaTeq vaccination: Evaluation from worldwide spontaneous reporting data using a self-controlled case series approach," *Vaccine*, January 14, 2015, https://doi .org/10.1016/j.vaccine.2015.01.005.

[45] Oregon Medical Board, "Order of Emergency Suspension."

[46] Centers for Disease Control and Prevention, "General Recommendations on Immunization: Recommendations of the Advisory Committee on Immunization Practices (ACIP) and the American Academy of Family Physicians (AAFP)," *MMWR*, February 8, 2002, https://www.cdc.gov/mmwr/preview/mmwrhtml/rr5102a1.htm.

[47] Oregon Health Authority, "Exemptions and Immunity," *Oregon.gov*, accessed February 23, 2021, https://www.oregon.gov/oha/PH/PreventionWellness/VaccinesImmunization /GettingImmunized/Pages/SchExemption.aspx. Archived at https://web.archive .org/web/20210223201256/https://www.oregon.gov/oha/PH/PreventionWellness /VaccinesImmunization/GettingImmunized/Pages/SchExemption.aspx.

48 Oregon Administrative Rules, Chapter 333, Division 50, *Oregon State Archives*, accessed February 23, 2021, https://secure.sos.state.or.us/oard/displayDivisionRules .action?selectedDivision=1265. See: Rule 0050, "Immunization Requirements" (OAR 333-050-0050).

49 OAR 333-050-0020.

50 OAR 333-050-0050.

What Dr. Paul's Patient Data Tell Us about the Health of Unvaccinated Children

1 Lyons-Weiler and Thomas, "Relative Incidence of Office Visits."

2 Ibid.

3 For a helpful explanation of the difference, see: Audrey Schnell, "The Difference Between Relative Risk and Odds Ratios," *The Analysis Factor*, accessed March 3, 2021, https://www.theanalysisfactor.com/the-difference-between-relative-risk-and-odds -ratios/. In short, the odds ratio calculation involves dividing the number of diagnoses in a cohort into the number of nondiagnosed patients, whereas relative risk involves diving the same numerator into the total number of patients in the cohort.

4 There are several errors in this section of the paper. The reported rate of diagnosis among the vaccinated and unvaccinated were respectively presented as "7/2647 (0.00264)" and "34/561 (0.0499)". These calculations should be 7/2,763 (0.0025) and 34/561 (0.0606), respectively. The odds ratio is presented as 0.054. This should be 0.039: (7/2,756) ÷ (34/527). The relative risk is presented as 0.053. This should be 0.042: (7/2,763) ÷ (34/561). The number needed to treat (NNT), which in this case is the number needed to vaccinate, is presented as 21.15. This should be 17.22: 1 ÷ (0.0606 - 0.0025). Dr. Lyons-Weiler has published a correction: Dr. James Lyons-Weiler, "Erratum: Lyons-Weiler and Thomas (2020)," *JamesLyonsWeiler.com*, March 4, 2021, https://jameslyonsweiler.com/2021/03/04/erratum-re-lyons-weiler-and-thomas-2020/.

5 Matthew J. Maenner et al., "Prevalence of Autism Spectrum Disorder Among Children Aged 8 Years—Autism and Developmental Disabilities Monitoring Network, 11 Sites, United States, 2016," *MMWR Surveillance Summaries*, March 27, 2020, http:// dx.doi.org/10.15585/mmwr.ss6904a1.

6 Lyons-Weiler and Thomas, "Relative Incidence of Office Visits"; Lyons-Weiler and Thomas, "Correction."

7 Centers for Disease Control and Prevention, "Data and Statistics About ADHD," *CDC .gov*, last reviewed November 16, 2020, accessed March 4, 2021, https://www.cdc.gov /ncbddd/adhd/data.html. Archived at https://web.archive.org/web/20210304205026 /https://www.cdc.gov/ncbddd/adhd/data.html.

8 Lyons-Weiler and Thomas, "Relative Incidence of Office Visits."

Conclusion

1 Laura Karas, "During the COVID-19 Pandemic, the Opioid Epidemic Continues," *Bill of Health*, Petrie-Flom Center at Harvard Law School, November 6, 2020, https:// blog.petrieflom.law.harvard.edu/2020/11/06/covid-pandemic-opioid-epidemic/;

Art Van Zee, "The Promotion and Marketing of OxyContin: Commercial Triumph, Public Health Tragedy," *American Journal of Public Health*, February 2009, https://www.ncbi.nlm.nih.gov/pmc/articles/PMC2622774/.

2   Senate Bill 254, 81st Oregon Legislative Assembly, 2021 Regular Session, Introduced January 11, 2021, https://olis.oregonlegislature.gov/liz/2021R1/Measures/Overview /SB254. For date of introduction, see also: https://legiscan.com/OR/bill/SB254/2021.